THE PILGRIM'S PLAN

For Optimal Health, Abundant Energy And Living Lean Without Prescriptions!

Dennis Burge

Cover design, text and internal layout by Ken Burge and A. McCollum

This publication is designed to provide accurate information in regard to the subject matter covered. It is sold with the understanding that both the author and publisher are not engaged in rendering legal, accounting, medical, or other professional services. If professional services in any of these areas of expertise are required, the services of a competent professional person should be sought.

Special thanks to Ken Burge, Archion Consulting, LLC.

Printed by Litho Printers & Bindery Cassville, MO 65625 *www. printlitho.com*

ISBN 978-1-5323-7358-9

Distribution—Pilgrim's Plan, LLC. *www.pilgrimsplan.com*

Facebook:
Community of Pilgrims dedicated to the Christian Keto Community
https://www.facebook.com/groups/communityofpilgrims/

Second Edition
10 9 8 7 6 5 4 3 2 1

THIS BOOK IS FOR YOU IF...

If you are currently suffering from any of the **five major signs of metabolic syndrome**...then this book is especially for you! Here they are listed so you can be sure this book is for you!

The Five Signs Of Metabolic Syndrome

1. If you have high blood pressure of 135/85mm Hg or greater, this book will resolve your problem without prescription drugs!

2. If you have high-fasting blood sugar of 125 mg/dl or higher, this book will teach you how to keep it under 100 mg/dl, thus preventing Type II Diabetes.

3. If you have low good cholesterol (HDL), defined for men as less than 40 mg/dl or for women less than 50 mg/dl, then this book will show you how to increase it to healthy levels!

4. If you have high triglycerides, the number one indicator of cardiovascular disease, of 150 mg/dl or higher, then this book will explain how to keep it under 100 mg/dl, thus protecting you from the ravages of cardiovascular disease!

5. If you have a large waist size of 40 inches or larger for men or 35 inches for women, then this book will reveal to you how to win the battle of the bulge once and for all!

THIS BOOK IS ALSO FOR YOU IF YOU ARE JUST SICK AND TIRED OF BEING SICK AND TIRED.

Who will benefit from ketosis? People who are overweight, have type 1 and 2 diabetes, cancer, leukemia, heart disease, any neurological disorder (including epilepsy, Parkinson, Alzheimer, MS or multiple sclerosis, senile dementia, schizophrenia, and depression), any digestive disorder (including IBD or Crohn's disease and ulcerative colitis, gastritis, IBS, liver cirrhosis, and hepatitis), any respiratory problem (asthma, bronchitis, COPD, emphysema, etc.) and any other inflammatory condition - or about 90% of overall population.

Do you long for energy you once possessed in your younger years? Maybe you've gained some extra weight in the recent years and nothing you have tried has worked to remove it. Perhaps your cognitive powers have declined and your memories of peoples' names, places, and events in your life are difficult to recall.

This book is for you if you want to learn how to lose fat with no hunger and cravings, while at the same time increasing energy and mental clarity. You will thank me once you have read this book and applied its principles. I promise.

Table of Contents

MEDICAL DISCLAIMER

This book is presented solely for motivational and informational purpose, and is not intended to be a substitute for a consultation with a licensed, healthcare practitioner.

If you are using prescription medicine, do not discontinue its use.

Tell your doctor about your plans to adopt the Pilgrim's Plan way of eating.

Ask your doctor to work with you on this and to adjust your medication accordingly.

Be patient, no pun intended. It will take a little time before you are able to be prescription drug free.

If your doctor is unwilling to help you reach your goal through the nutritional guidelines contained in this book, this reveals two unfortunate realities about your doctor.

First, he or she is committed to the pharmaceutical industry and believes their drugs are the only solution to your problem.

Second, it reveals a lack of knowledge concerning the healing properties of food.

This is very common among doctors today because they have little or no true nutritional education. This is unfortunate, indeed, in light of Hippocrates's famous quote, "Let food be your medicine, let medicine be your food."

Free yourself from such a doctor or you will be on prescription drugs for the rest of your life.

Seek out a doctor who is willing to help and encourage you on your journey to optimal health.

Pilgrims, please do not read into this disclaimer that I am anti-doctors or hospitals. I am not!

We have the best doctors and nurses in the world today. I believe they are doing the best they know how to preserve life.

If it were not for them, I would not be here today. I have had two emergency surgeries in my life.

One was for an inflamed and swollen appendix when I was 10 years old and the other was the removal of my gallbladder when I was 60 years old.

The doctor in both cases said I was only a day or maybe two from life-threatening circumstances! I am very thankful to the good Lord above and those doctors and their staff who saved my life!

MEDICAL EXPERT QUOTES THAT SUPPORT THE PRINCIPLES IN THE PILGRIM'S PLAN

"The best diet for overall health, and specifically for the heart, brain, and cancer risk reduction, is a diet that's aggressively low in carbohydrates with an abundance of healthful fat…."
Dr. David Perlmutter

"The low fat diet has been one of the biggest disasters in modern medicine, and in my view has fueled the obesity epidemic. It's time we stopped counting calories and eat real food."
Dr. Aseem Malhotra

"Processed food causes metabolic syndrome."
Dr. Robert Lustig

"Your health and lifespan will mostly be determined by the proportion of fat vs. sugar you burn in a lifetime."
Dr. Ron Rosedale

"It is clear to me that a low carbohydrate diet is the safest change you can make. You know this because after 40 years of an obsessive/compulsive effort by the medical establishment trying to find something wrong [with low carb diet] and 40 years of the press begging for a scare story…they've got nothing. "
Dr. Richard Feinman

"Ketosis deals effectively with all the problems of a diet rich in carbs – the one recommended by mainstream science. It is a crime to discourage the consumption of a high fat diet, considering that a ketogenic diet shrinks tumors in human and animal models, and enhances our brain's resilience against stress and toxicity."
Dr. Gabriela Segura

"The doctor of the future will give no medicine but will interest his patients in the care of the human frame in diet and in the cause and prevention of disease."
Thomas Edison

DEDICATION

I dedicate this book to my son Ken and my wife Patty.

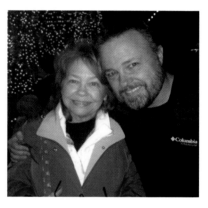 Without Ken's Christmas gift given to me seven years ago, a book about regaining one's health, I probably would not be here today.

The good Lord above and the knowledge contained in that book saved my life.

As I opened my eyes to the truth that this health-related book offered, it unlocked a desire and passion inside me to know exactly how my God-given body could be restored to optimal health.

It was Patty, though, who insisted I visit a local health fair where I learned I was in danger of a stroke or heart attack.

My gratitude for Ken's gift and Patty's wisdom is limitless.

Because of their deep love and concern for me and their desire to see me regain my health, I am not only alive today, but I am thriving.

I want to also dedicate this book to every brother and sister in the body of Christ and especially their pastors who are struggling with health issues.

ACKNOWLEDGMENTS

I am very thankful for my wonderful wife, Patty, who did the final editing of this book. Her knowledge of grammar and keen eye has made this book one we are both very proud of!

Thank you Bubba aka Shortcake.

I also want to thank Larry Quinalty, Ed. D. for his expertise in helping edit the grammar of this book.

A special thanks goes to Marty Jenkins and Amanda Mc-Collum at Litho Printers and Bindery for their excellent advice and suggestions in producing this book.

INTRODUCTION

Greetings Pilgrims!

I'm Pastor Dennis Burge and for 18 years I've served as the pastor of Calvary Chapel Church of Monett, Missouri.

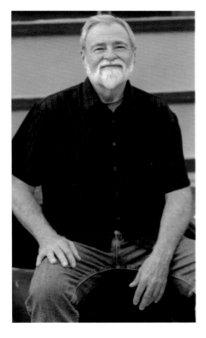

This book details the remarkable story of how I was able to lose eighty pounds of debilitating fat and enjoy optimal health, abundant energy, and living lean without prescription drugs!

Remember, my story is just my story. I am not a doctor, nor do I pretend to be.

My experience and results that I share in this book are supported by thousands of other pilgrims who have also achieved optimal health and prescription-free living.

This book teaches valuable lessons which are both profound in their simplicity and effectiveness.

This book outlines a way of eating and living that our great-grandparents would recognize, but many of us have forgotten.

This book is also a resounding rejection of the Standard American Diet (SAD). What an apt acronym! The conventional wisdom of the establishment has failed miserably.

I am a firm believer that in order to move forward, we must go back to the basics and take charge of our own health.

My aim is to keep this book short and simple. I could have easily written 300 pages, but who has time for that? I am using less words and sharing what I have learned since I began this journey six years ago?

You can easily read this book and implement my strategies within days. You will be amazed at how quickly you experience a positive change.

You will also be amazed to discover you never have to restrict calories, count calories, weigh anything, or go hungry! Your meals will be nutritious, delicious, and satisfying.

What Is A Pilgrim?

You may be wondering why I call myself a pilgrim, and why I refer to people as Pilgrims who follow the teachings in this book.

**A pilgrim is someone on a journey
with the intent of improving their life.**

As a thirteen-year-old boy, I was introduced to Pilgrim's Progress, the number one Christian devotional book of all time. In this book, John Bunyan takes the reader on a journey from the City of Destruction to Heaven. I've always liked the idea of being a Pilgrim on life's journey. Because I was on a journey to regain my health I started calling myself a Pilgrim along with others I was able to teach.

My own pilgrimage was truly a matter of life and death! I could have chosen to live a life dependent upon prescription drugs with all their horrible side effects. I chose to live the abundant life Jesus spoke of in John 10:10.

Jesus also said, "And you shall know the truth, and the truth shall make you free" (John 8:32, NKJV). Well, praise the Lord, I discovered the truth that would set me free from having to use prescriptions drugs. Now, I am enjoying the abundant life Jesus promised.

Let's Get Started!
I'm excited for you as you embark on this journey!

Through it all, I will be here for you. I am ready to lend a hand, answer questions, and help motivate and inspire you to reach optimal health and vitality.

Dennis Burge

Pastor Dennis Burge
Calvary Chapel Of Monett
Monett, Missouri

SECTION ONE:

HOW I LOST 80 POUNDS

AND REGAINED MY YOUTH

CHAPTER ONE

MY PURPOSE

"I will proclaim what the Lord has done"
(Psalm 118:17, NIV).

For many years I have faithfully taught God's word and proclaimed the gospel of Christ while discipling those who have received Him as their Lord and Savior. By God's grace I will continue to do this as long as I am able. After all, there is no higher calling and mission in life than that of being a servant of God!

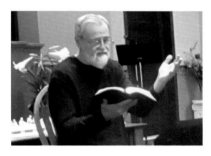

"The fruit of the righteous is a tree of life, and he who wins souls is wise"
(Proverbs 11:30, NKJV).

Where a man or woman will spend eternity is of far greater importance than the brief time we spend in our earthly bodies. Therefore fulfilling my pastoral duties is of paramount importance to me.

While living in these earthly bodies our good Lord created, we owe it to Him and ourselves to take care of them so we may live in optimal health and reflect His glory.

When we are at peak and optimal health, we are able to serve God with more energy, vigor, creativity, and endurance than if we are sick, hobbled, or so tired we can't get off the couch.

We were made in the image and likeness of God (see Genesis 1:27). He created Adam and Eve in perfect health. There was no sickness or disease of any kind. They lived, and breathed, and walked in divine health.

Yes, they eventually died because, "For the wages of sin is death" (Romans 6:23, NKJV).

However, I do not believe they died sick or diseased. I believe they died of old age.

After the fall, there was an expiration date for every man (see Hebrews 9:27). For some it was 70 years, for others 80, and some perhaps as many as 120 (see Genesis 6:3 and Psalm 90:10).

Remember when Moses left this earth at 120 years old, the Bible says, "yet his eyesight was perfect and he was as strong as a young man" (Deuteronomy 34:7, The Living Bible).

Learn To Truly Live
What I have learned in the last six years is that I can live—and I mean really live—all the days of my life!

Don't believe for a minute that it is just normal to be sick and tired the last half of your life. It is not normal, and everyone must reject that notion.

It has been said that some men die when they are 40. They just don't bury them until they are 80. This statement may be true, but, what a shame!

Those last 40 years, men are kept alive with prescription drugs and all their horrible side effects.

Did you know that in 2011, doctors wrote 4.02 billion drug prescriptions according to the journal *ACS Chemical Neuroscience?*

Pilgrims, that is not living. That's a horror movie worse than anything Hollywood has produced.

My Personal Health Crisis

Just a few short years ago, I faced a major health crisis and the reality of an impending stroke. I had to figure out how to change my diet and reclaim my God-given health and fitness.

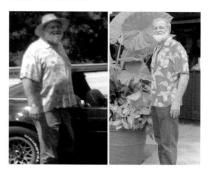

Over the course of just ten months, I lost 80 pounds of debilitating fat and gained amazing amounts of energy, endurance, and a new found zest for a life with no limitations!

The next chapter will share more details of my transformation, and I want you to realize that you can do the same.

Perhaps you are thinking my transformation was a fluke, something so rare it could never happen to you.

While I can admit it was miraculous, it was the kind of miracle that is common to those who adopt this way of eating. I am no outlier. You can achieve the same result. Jesus

said, "I have come that they may have life, and that they might have it more abundantly" (John 10:10, NKJV).
I believe that is not only true spiritually, but also physically.

By following my example and implementing the strategies in this book, you will be amazed at the benefits you will begin to experience:

Here are some of those benefits:

1. Effortless weight loss, especially belly fat, as your body learns to burn fat.

2. No more Carb-Coma — this plan eliminates the roller-coaster ride by design.

3. You'll experience a dramatic increase in energy with a steady release all day long.

4. Naturally lowers your blood sugar, thereby preventing Type II Diabetes.

5. Naturally lowers your blood pressure, guarding against stroke and heart attack.

6. Naturally lowers your triglycerides, the major indicator of cardiovascular disease.

7. Good cholesterol (HDL) will increase…vital for proper hormonal balance.

8. Your mental clarity will immensely improve. Brain fog will go away and memory will significantly improve.

9. No more digestive issues such as bloating, heartburn, constipation, or diarrhea!

My Commission

My commission now is to "go into all the world" (see Mark 16:15 NKJV) through every available means, teaching people not only how to have eternal life, but how they can live in optimal health and fulfill God's plan for their lives here on Earth!

Pilgrims, the Apostle Paul shared with us in First Corinthians 12:8-10 that there are nine spiritual gifts.

The only gifts I have ever asked God for is "the word of wisdom and the word of knowledge" (1 Corinthians 12:8, KJV).

I believe this book is the answer to that prayer, and what a joy it is to share with you the wisdom and knowledge I have been given.

My gratitude is immense, and I feel as if I owe an enormous debt to help as many as possible to receive the same life extension that I have.

Pilgrims, my prayer for you is the one John the Apostle prayed for his friend, Gaius.

"Beloved, I pray that you may prosper in all things and be in health, just as your soul prospers" (3 John 1:2, NKJV).

In Chapter Two, I want to share with you my own personal health transformation so you can learn from my journey and hopefully avoid the life-threatening situation I experienced.

This is my son Ken and me after our Keto transformation. The young man in the background is my grandson T.J. who also has adopted a Keto way of life and is a lean mean fat burning machine!

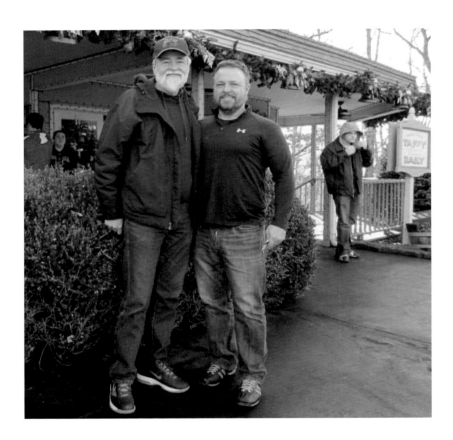

CHAPTER TWO

IN THE BEGINNING

"In the beginning God created the heavens and the Earth"
(Genesis 1:1, NKJV).

My journey began on Christmas day, 2011. My oldest son, Ken, handed me a gift: a book about how to transform one's life and enjoy optimal health.

In all honesty, I wasn't thrilled about it, but I knew why Ken had given it to me. Being 64 years old, I was obese and very tired. The worst part was that I was in danger of having a stroke or heart attack and didn't even know it.

Two months and a trip to the hospital passed before I read the book.

On the verge of a stroke
It was a cold day at the end of February 2012 when my wife insisted I go with her to a health fair being held at our local hospital.

Of course, I didn't want to go. A lot of pastors and grand-pas my age are overweight. I thought I was pretty normal.

I will admit, it did bother me a bit when little children would stare at me, tug on their mom's sleeve, and insist I was Santa Claus. To be fair, I did have a white beard to go along with the big belly!

That day at the hospital marked the beginning of my journey back to health.

The nurse measured my height and then weighed me. I was 6 feet tall and weighed 253 pounds. My Body Mass Index (BMI) was 34—clinically obese.

Unfortunately, that wasn't all.

My blood sample revealed I was on the cusp of having full-blown Type II diabetes. My blood glucose reading was 125 mg/dl. Doctors prescribe medication at 126 mg/dl; usually Metformin, insulin or both.

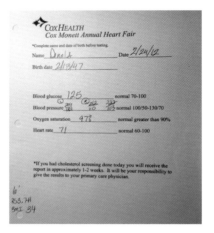

My grandmother had lost a leg due to diabetes. I vividly remember my mother giving her insulin shots before she passed away. How sad to lose a leg and have to be stuck with a needle everyday for the rest of one's life.

It appeared that I was facing the same destiny.

Worse still, the nurse took my blood pressure, paused, and said, "Let me check it again, sir." She then left to find the head nurse, who said, "Mr. Burge, come with me down the hall to a quiet room and rest a while."

Ten minutes later, she returned and checked my blood pressure for a third time. The first reading was 204/101.

The second was 212/110. Now it was 222/103. She explained I was in imminent danger of having a stroke or heart attack.

She suggested I immediately ask my doctor for blood pressure medication. I told her I would discuss it with my wife, and we would pray about it. The nurse didn't know I did not have a doctor.

After praying and thinking deeply about the nurse's comment, I didn't feel led to go to a doctor. I didn't want to become dependent on prescription drugs for the rest of my life.

Instead, I opened the book my son Ken had given me and began reading.

Over the years, I had read several books, magazine articles, and had seen thousands of television commercials regarding health and diet.

However, this book was very different from anything I had read before.

In it, the conventional wisdom of the medical establishment, as it relates to a proper diet, was turned upside-down.

My Epiphany
The book made me ask some very important questions.

If conventional health wisdom was right, why are hospitals full?

Why are two-thirds of the adult population over-weight, and why are one-third of those people obese?

Why has childhood obesity in this country nearly tripled since 1980?

Why is the Type II Diabetes pandemic spreading all over the world?

Why is heart disease and cancer still the two leading causes of death?

As I pondered these sobering facts, I began to trust this book and take its advice on how to regain my health through proper diet and avoid the side effects of prescription drugs.

I devoured that book and have since then purchased more than eighty books of its kind. I wanted to thoroughly understand this subject and validate the veracity of the book my son had given me.

I spent over a thousand dollars purchasing those books. I have read them as well as having spent hundreds of hours researching this subject via the internet.

The results I have achieved in terms of transforming my own health and fitness levels have been nothing short of amazing and well worth my investment!

However, you need not spend a thousand dollars to achieve what I have.

I ask you to just trust me and follow the simple plan outlined in this book.

You will achieve what I have and perhaps more!

The first thing I decided to do to reclaim my health might shock you!

I began by suspending my membership at the local YMCA!

I know my action was unconventional. I did so because of my extreme high risk for stroke or heart attack. Exercise served only to exhaust me and then ramp up my appetite. I would overeat and lose any benefit I might have gained. So, I made a decision to lose 80 pounds of fat. Afterwards I rejoined the YMCA and to this day, I maintain my weight loss through aerobic and anaerobic exercise.

Next, I decided to concentrate all my effort into learning about how to achieve optimal health through scientifical-ly-based nutrition strategies.

Positive results came almost immediately. I began to lose, on average, two pounds per week. Experts agree this is a healthy and realistic goal!

One year later I re-joined the YMCA. On that February day in 2013, I weighed 173 pounds and had an abundance of energy to burn! One year had passed since that fateful day at the hospital, and I had regained my health. I had never felt better in my life!

As a boy, my passion was basketball. But, it had been over 40 years since I had played full-court competition ball.

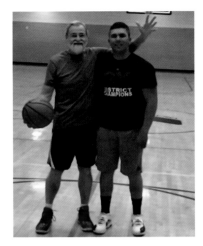

As hard as it is for most people to imagine, I now play three to four times per week with a group of men half my age. Some of them like Kyle could be my grandsons!

Can someone say, "Praise the Lord?"

In August 2013, our local hospital hosted another health fair. I was anxious to go back and reassess my basic health stats after losing 80 pounds.

Now my BMI was 23 and my resting heart rate had dropped from 71 to 57 beats per minute. My cholesterol total was 165. My HDL was 72 and the LDL was 86. My triglyceride reading was 37. I was clearly no longer in danger of a stroke or heart attack.

A few weeks after the health fair, I ran my first 5K race. Notice I said *ran*, not walked! Pilgrims, I had never run three miles in my life. This was a first for me!

Gone were my high blood pressure, blood sugar/ glucose issues, as well as 80 pounds of fat. The heartburn I had tolerated for many years was gone. I used to always keep plenty of Rolaids in my car, bedroom and my pockets. I struggled with constipation and diarrhea for most of my adult life, but now that was gone too.

In recent years, I had even begun to struggle to remember people's names and was embarrassed when I ran into an old classmate. Sometimes I couldn't remember names of people with whom I used to work. It was so frustrating to not be able to recall the names of people from my past!

But now, when I meet old friends, names quickly come to mind!

This is a testament to the body's ability to heal itself, if it is given the right nutrients.

My family was very thankful for the miraculous transformation in my health.

Praise the Lord!

My miraculous transformation took place in the last ten months of 2012.

The most meaningful thing to note is that I have effortlessly maintained my weight and health to this day!

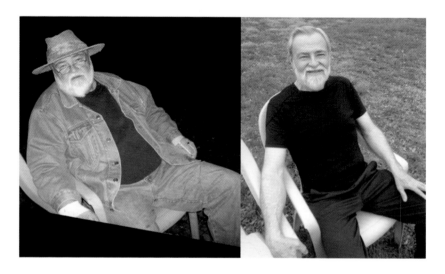

**The Pilgrim's Plan is a lifestyle, and
a lifestyle that is sustainable for the rest of your life!**

I never counted calories or weighed anything, and I never went hungry.

I thank the good Lord above, my son, and my wife for saving my life.

That Christmas gift turned out to be the best gift I have ever received, and this book, the culmination of all I have learned, is my way of paying it forward to as many people as I can.

I'm excited for you because the next chapter lays out a roadmap for you to follow.

If you follow this roadmap, the reward at the end of your journey will be your ideal body.

The road isn't that long, and it isn't that hard either.

However, it does require that you begin.

So, let's get started!

CHAPTER THREE

THE JOURNEY AHEAD...

"Where there is no vision, the people perish..."
(Proverbs 29:18, KJV).

Let me give you a taste of how the rest of this book is laid out, and how I recommend that you learn and implement the wisdom on these pages.

The Pilgrim's Plan contains six sections, plus an additional four appendixes.

I will give you a sneak peak at each section so that you can better understand the organization of this book.

Section One: How I Lost 80 Pounds And Regained My Youth

This is the current section you are reading. In this section, I've been sharing with you how the Pilgrim's Plan came to be, my own personal health crisis, and this brief overview chapter of the book itself.

Section Two: Dispelling Myths

This section helps prepare you for the journey ahead by addressing some of the prevailing myths you may have about health and nutrition. It is important to talk about the broad misconceptions that govern our daily choices and why our nation, according to the C.D.C. says 70.7 percent of adults overweight. Of that 70.7 percent, 37.9 percent are classified as obese.

Section Three: Leveraging Real Food For Natural Fat Loss

This section is all about explaining the core concepts of the Pilgrim's Plan. I'll be showing you how eating only natural unprocessed God-given food and eliminating food groups that challenge digestion can dramatically improve your health within days. This step will improve your overall health and restore proper digestion and elimination, while also providing you with all the minerals and vitamins your body needs as it rebuilds your health one cell at a time. This forms the foundation of the Pilgrim's Plan.

Section Four: Turbocharging Your Fat Loss

In section four you'll learn how to enter nutritional (or dietary) ketosis so that your body will draw upon stored fat for energy. Have you ever heard the saying "melt away fat"? You'll experience it. Initially, you can expect to lose three to four pounds per week while in ketosis. The weight loss will slow as you come within striking range of your ideal weight, but you will continue to lose weight as long as you stay in nutritional ketosis. You will also explore the benefits of intermittent fasting and how it can deliver many health benefits. You will find the benefits of this natural rhythm of eating are legendary, and you'll be shocked at how easy it is to implement. Don't worry, you will still be eating plenty of food. We'll adjust your eating times, so that you achieve some spectacular results.

Section Five: Lifestyle Changes For Optimal Fat Loss

We will review several lifestyle adjustments in this section that can dramatically increase your body's ability to burn fat and reach optimal levels of health. In addition, I will review the role exercise and activity played in my journey to optimal health, as well as a few other important factors that impact weight loss. You may be shocked at how little exercise you need to enjoy its benefits. But in fact, you will find your new energy level inspires you to be much more active than you ever imagined!

Section Six: The Master Key

One of the most important parts of the Pilgrim's Plan is contained in section six. I'll be helping you learn how to create a very strong vision for your future health, along with the tools to ensure what you envision becomes reality. During this step you will learn the motivational secrets that will allow you to reach your goals. You can live with more energy, a lean body, and much more vigor. Next, I will ask you to take your commitment to living the Pilgrim's Plan way to the next level by sharing this plan with others through a variety of methods. I want you to become a vessel to help others, just as you needed help before you went through the Pilgrim's Plan.

Appendixes

I have assembled four excellent appendixes in this book that you will find very helpful on your journey back to optimal health. I have condensed some of my best advice, recommendations, and lists into a few easy to read pages in these appendixes.

Summary

These simple six sections of the book (plus four Appendixes) will guide you to optimal health and well-being. Once I discovered how to implement the truths found in these pages, my health began improving immediately and dramatically.

Now that you understand the six phases of the Pilgrim's Plan, let's move on to Section Two and start dispelling some common myths related to health and fat loss. This next chapter will look at how we, as a nation, were led astray in terms of our health.

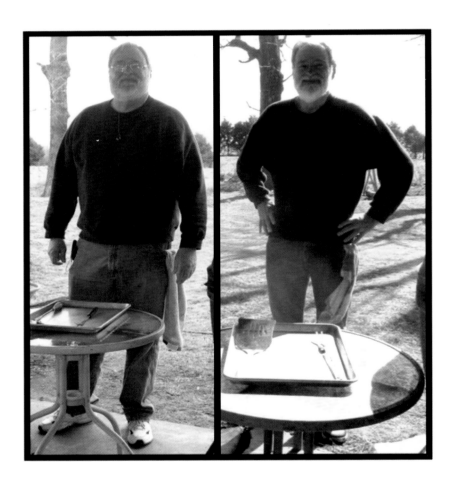

SECTION TWO:

DISPELLING MYTHS

CHAPTER FOUR

HOW WE BECAME THE FATTEST NATION ON EARTH

"Wisdom is shown to be right by its results"
(Matthew 11:19, NLT).

Pilgrims, did you know that during the last 40 years in the United States there has been a dramatic rise in obesity, Type II Diabetes, heart disease, cancer, and Alzheimer's?

This chapter explains how these startling facts are the direct result of us following the infamous food pyramid promoted by our government back in the late 1970s.

When it comes to dietary wisdom, the wise guys of our age have failed us miserably!

We know that the first four recorded heart attacks in America were in 1912, according to the journal of the American Medical Association (AMA). Since then, with the dramatic increase in starchy carbohydrate consumption and processed foods, we've seen a dramatic rise in the following diseases.

- Heart Disease
- Cancer
- Type II Diabetes
- Stroke
- Alzheimer's Disease
- Obesity — a hormonal disease

A few interesting facts about this list:

- Did you know that heart disease is still the number one cause of death in America?

- Tragically, a new case of Alzheimer's Disease is diagnosed every 65 seconds! Many medical professionals now believe this is actually the third leading cause of death in seniors!

The Flawed Food Pyramid

We were told in the 1970's that a diet high in starchy carbohydrates, low in fat, and moderate in proteins is healthy. Now multiple studies have confirmed that this advice has been devastating to the health of this nation and the world.

We were told animal fat was the cause of cardiovascular disease and the alarming increase of overweight and obese people in our nation.

70.7 percent of Americans are now considered overweight, and of that group, 37.9 percent of them are considered clinically obese.

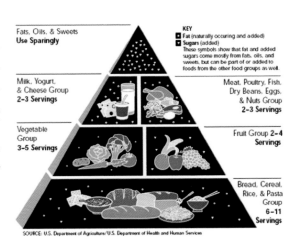

SOURCE: U.S. Department of Agriculture/U.S. Department of Health and Human Services

The latest surveys show that one-third of our children are overweight.

Due to these misguided recommendations, obesity has doubled in this generation and cardiovascular disease is still the number one cause of death in America.

Cancer is second on this list, followed by stroke.

Alzheimer's is now being called "Type III Diabetes" because it has, at its root, the same cause as Type II Diabetes. This insulin resistance is caused by the overconsumption of processed carbohydrates.

Along with the weight gain has come a pandemic of **Type II Diabetes,** which **doubles the risk of Alzheimer's disease.**

Type II Diabetes was originally thought only to occur in adults, but this theory has been busted! Sadly, our country now has an alarming number of children with Type II Diabetes.

Non-Alcohol Fatty Liver Disease
Between 60 and 90 million people have non-alcoholic fatty liver disease. High fructose corn syrup is the major contributor to this disease in adults as well as children, via the sugary drinks we consume at record levels!

I mention these facts to illustrate the simple point that the health crisis in this country is at a breaking point.

There has been a massive decline in the health of Americans since low fat, high carb dietary recommendations became national policy, promoted by our government back in the 1970's.

We spend more money than all the other developed countries in the world on health care, and yet we are the fattest and the sickest.

The food pyramid, promoted by our government, has resulted in the health crisis we are experiencing today. I would like to tell you that these guidelines were based upon verifiable scientific research.

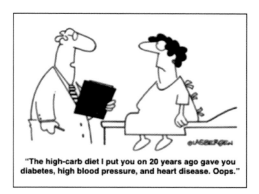

"The high-carb diet I put you on 20 years ago gave you diabetes, high blood pressure, and heart disease. Oops."

Unfortunately, it was not! Our hospitals are filled with millions of people suffering from the result of this epic-failed experiment. Only God knows how many have died as a result of it!

The real tragedy is that information was available that would have led to a different food pyramid than the one we have.

In 1863, a man named William Banting published the "Letter On Corpulence" which was addressed to the public. He described how he lost 50 pounds and regained his health.

His approach to losing fat was the very same principles outlined in this book.

Banting had fought his weight problem all his adult life. He had tried eating less and exercising more. He tried everything any doctor of his day would advise, including taking Turkish baths. His efforts were to no avail.

He finally met a doctor named William Harvey. Harvey had recently heard a lecture given by Claude Bernard, who had discovered that the body, via the liver, could produce its own glucose through a process called gluco-neogenesis without any carbohydrate ingestion!

This lead him to suggest to Banting that he try a carbohy-drate restricted diet, and see if he could shed those extra pounds.

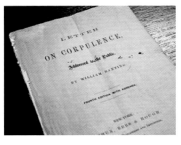

He had found the key that would unlock his fat stores, and it required no exercise!

Banting's experiment proved that a low carbohydrate, plus high fat diet (LCHF) would result in weight loss!

He sold more than 50,000 copies of his "letter" on the streets of London and helped thousands of others win the war of obesity and regain their health.

Mr. Banting was 64 years old when he began this way of eating and lived another 17 years in good health before his passing at the age of 81!

Unfortunately, the medical establishment of his day did not promote his diet, and Banting's methods were set aside in favor of the conventional wisdom of the day. Afterall, Banting was not a doctor or a scientist, and there were no long-term studies to prove its benefits. The food industry realized that producing foods high in carbohydrates was much more economically profitable than promoting a diet high in animal products.

Then, in the 1960's, we were further lead astray due to the flawed and fraudulent diet hypothesis of a scientist named Dr. Ancel Keys.

Keys looked at six countries that had very little cardiovascular disease. At that time, cardiovascular disease was, and still is, the number one cause of death in America.

The diet of those six countries was predominantly starchy carbohydrates, some protein, and very little fat.

However, he did not reveal that his study also included 16 other countries that contradicted his conclusions.

His cherry-picked conclusions led to the infamous food pyramid, which recommended our diet consist of 55-60 percent of starchy carbohydrates, and no more than 30 percent fat with the rest in protein.

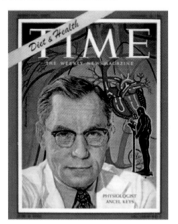

The results, not only in America but worldwide, have been devastating to the health of mankind.

Consider this: One in every 4,000 (0.00025 percent) people was diabetic in the late 1800s.

Today, 1,000 in every 4,000 (25 percent) are diabetic or pre-diabetic, and it is estimated that soon these numbers will rise to one in three men and two out of four women.

It doesn't take a rocket scientist to see the correlation.

Even with the bad news, there is hope.

Today, we know that a low carbohydrate diet, which is high in fat and moderate in protein, results in a lean, healthy body for those who are overweight.

Studies have shown that Type II Diabetics can eliminate their need for medication by eating a diet higher in healthy fats. I will teach you how to do this in my book!

One in every three adults in America has **high blood pressure, the silent killer.** I was one of them!

Pilgrims, follow the path outlined in this book and your blood pressure will normalize, and you will win the battle of the bulge too!

Preventing Diet Failure

People fail calorie restricted diets or excessive exercise programs because they are not sustainable for the long term. Science has shown that those who lose weight through caloric restriction almost always gain it back, and then some. Excessive exercise leads to adrenal fatigue, injury, as well as a ravenous appetite

The Pilgrim's Plan is sustainable for life, because it is NOT focused on calorie restriction or excessive exercise!

You will always be full and satisfied, and you won't be burning calories through long, boring hours at the gym.

Calorie-restricted diets cause primarily water and muscle loss and leave the dieter weak and miserable. People on these kinds of diets are always "hangry", which means angry AND hungry!

These types of diets also slow one's metabolism making it very difficult to lose weight, even while restricting calories!

No one in their right mind stays on that kind of a diet very long.

Solomon said, "Wisdom is the principle thing, therefore get wisdom" (Proverbs 4:7, KJV). He also said, "Happy is the man that findeth wisdom, and the man that getteth understanding." (Proverbs 3:3, KJV). Because "Wisdom is more precious than rubies, and nothing you desire can compare with her" (Proverbs 8:11, NIV). Because, **"Through me (wisdom) your days will be many and years will be added to your life**, if you are wise, your wisdom will reward you; if you are a mocker, you alone will suffer" (Prov. 9:11-12, NIV).

Pilgrims…be wise and join me on this journey.

Chemicals In Our Food Are Poisoning Our Bodies

Pilgrims, we must do our own research about health and nutrition and do our best to **eat clean, natural, unprocessed foods.** We must listen to our bodies, especially when they are grumbling and trying to tell us something.

Treating symptoms of impending health issues with just another prescription drug is not the answer!

It has been said that Americans do not have a health care system, only a disease-management system.

It has also been said that common sense is not common. Both are true!

Overconsumption of Salt And Sugar In Processed Foods

Let's address the deadly combination of salt and sugar that is prevalent in so many processed foods today.

Sugar is addictive and salt/potassium ratio imbalance in processed food leads to high blood pressure.

Have you ever wondered why so many processed foods are full of sugar and salt?

When fat was labeled as the cause of modern diseases and removed from processed food, manufacturers had a huge problem. The food tasted terrible!

By adding copious amounts of salt and sugar, these manufactured foods tasted good again. This strategy worked, albeit at the expense of the health of the nation.

The pounds keep piling on until we learn to eat the Pilgrim's Way of eating!

I firmly believe being overweight is not the result of overeating or lack of exercise for the majority of those struggling with their weight. In other words, **obesity is not a moral issue** or a laziness issue.

Oh, I suppose there a few Cretans in our society (See Titus 1:12, NIV). But most people are not lazy gluttons, which is what is implied when we are told to just eat less and exercise more.

KEY POINT:
The real cause of obesity is hormonal dysfunction.

What caused our hormones to be out of balance?

Was it too much protein in our diet? No!

Was it too much fat in our diet? No!

Was it too many starchy carbohydrates in our diet? Yes!

Pilgrims, starchy carbohydrates drive insulin up and insulin drives excess carbohydrates, straight to our fat depots!

Did we really think that we could eat Franken-foods manufactured in laboratories and have better health than when we eat of the natural foods God has provided for us?

Foods such as vegetables grown from the ground, or fruit from a tree, or animals raised in their natural habitat free of stress will always provide superior nutrition for our bodies. This is how God designed us to be nourished!

Did we really think that we could fry our foods in hydrogenated trans fats (the worst kind of man-made fat) and not pay a price?

Did we really think we could eat food from boxes and cans loaded with chemical compounds that we cannot even pronounce, nor our bodies recognize, without suffering serious side effects?

Did we really think we could consume unlimited amounts of sugar?

God never intended for us to eat highly processed, genetically engineered foods of our day.

Ninety cents of every dollar of today's food budget is spent on processed foods that did not exist 100 years ago. As much as 80 percent of the food in today's grocery stores is highly-processed, manufactured foods. They are loaded with added sugar, sodium, and cancer-causing chemicals. Pilgrims, for the sake of your health, generally speaking, stay out of the middle aisles of the grocery store!

In order to lose fat we need to create a hormonal environment that encourages fat burning automatically.

Processed foods are overwhelming the body's ability to overcome them and eliminate them. Our plumbing is clogged. The toxic waste is bound up and backed up in us. It makes us sick and manifests itself in maladies that were not prevalent in our great-grandfather's day.

Hippocrates was right when he said, "All disease begins in the gut."

Oh, Mighty God, Lord Jesus Christ, help us to wise up and be careful what we put in our mouths. In Your infinite wisdom, power and love, you designed us perfectly and gave us herbs, nuts, seeds, fruit, and then you even gave us, after the flood, meat to eat (See Genesis 2:15-16, 9:1-4). Help us to have the wisdom to follow Your plan!

DEATH BY DIET

We are what we eat, and we are what we don't,
When told what to eat, some of us won't,
'Cause to eat butter and eggs and milk and salt,
We are told will bring life, to a crashing halt.

And yet the cultures that do, they don't have disease,
They eat all of these things, as much as they please,
One hundred times the Recommended Daily Allowance,
Exceeding the RDA by the pound, and not by the ounce.

And every element, God put on the good Earth,
Is consumed every day, for its nutritional worth,
And they also eat lots of vitamins and lots of minerals,
Garlic and onions, they're not young at their funerals.

Lots of butter and salt, at one hundred having tea,
Americans, we don't, and we barely make seventy,
All day in the sun with their lives is the trend,
Hippocrates was right; the sun's your best friend.

Yet these cultures have taught us "it's not what we eat,"
But that which we don't, without nutrition we're beat.
We grow old while we're young, with premature death,
Believing we're right, as we exhale our last breath.

This premature death caused by doctor's advice,
Should cause the world to pause, and start to think twice,
With drugs so expensive, and vitamins so thrifty,
The shame is, your doctor age's naire over fifty.

Drugs are man-made powders, chemicals that kill,
Vitamins and minerals are God's design, His will,
And the health of the world, will be filled with sorrow,
If the doctors today, don't become nutritionists tomorrow.

Robert R. Barefoot

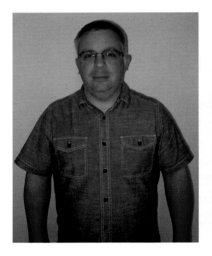 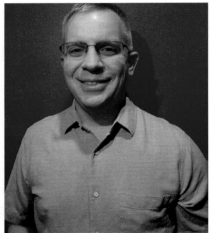

Michael Brittenham: Finally fog free!

My initial drive in changing the way I eat was simply to be healthier. I'd done all the normal things you do to lose weight but never felt healthy. I read the Pilgrim's Plan and realized there was another way. I had been out of shape and suffering from acid reflux since my early 20's. From the day I cut sugar and other carbs from my diet and started eating high fat I no longer suffer from acid reflux. I began to lose weight and more than anything I genuinely feel better. Over the first few weeks I thought this was simply a physical improvement.

But, then one day it was like someone flipped a switch and my mental clarity shot through the roof.

I was able to engage in conversations and meetings at work in a way I hadn't in years. Feeling good has been wonderful but the greatest benefit has been no longer living under a fog.

Michael Brittenham

CHAPTER FIVE

WHY WE ALL GOT FAT

"Man shall not live by bread alone…"
(Matthew 4:4, KJV).

Pilgrims, before I dive into the heart of this chapter, I would be remiss if I didn't provide you with a rudimentary understanding of how our food is really made up of three basic macronutrients. If you are like I was, you may have gone most of your life without paying much attention to some of these basics.

Nutrition 101

Every time you sit down to eat, no matter if it's a simple meal made at home, or a fancy meal at a restaurant, or even an apple from the orchard, the food you eat can be broken down into just three macronutrients. Not all foods have all three! Some foods are just made up of one or two of the macronutrients!

So what are the three basic macronutrients?

They are protein, fats, and carbohydrates.

That's it.

Protein is the basic building block of your muscles, hair, fingernails and the connective tissues of your body. **Protein is required for life.** Examples of the major foods that contain protein are all meats, fish, chicken, and dairy.

Fat (actually lipids) is critical to brain function, joint function, many chemical processes in your body, and **fat is required for life.** Examples of foods that provide healthy fats are eggs, avocados, coconut oil, olive oil, lard, tallow, butter, heavy cream, and nuts/seeds.

Of the three macronutrients, **only carbohydrates are not required for life.** There will be more on that later. Some foods that provide carbohydrates are all grain products, vegetables, legumes/beans, nuts, and fruit.

Carbohydrates are a component of many foods and are ultimately all broken down into glucose, which is a simple sugar the body can use for fuel.

The Calorie In/Calorie Out Myth

The medical establishment has told us that we gain weight when we fail to burn the calories that we consume on a daily basis.

The acronym for this Calories In/Calories Out myth is CICO and indeed it is PSYCHO!

The truth is, consuming more calories in a day than you burn does not technically make you fat: instead it's your inability to access and burn the fat stored on your body that keeps you fat!

KEY POINT:
Pilgrims, a major key to fat loss is to turn on your body's natural ability to burn stored fat.

Consider this illustration of homeostasis, which is your body's ability to naturally balance energy intake and expenditure.

In a recent experiment, a young man named Sam Feltham was given 5,800 calories per day for 21 days. This was 2300 calories above his normal 3500 calories per day. The diet was essentially the one described in this book. If all calories are the same, as the medical community says they are, he should have gained 13 pounds. He did not! He gained three pounds.

Later, they tried it again. This time he was given a high carbohydrate, low fat, moderate protein diet totaling 5,800 calories.

He gained 15 pounds in 21 days!

The medical community was about right when he was eating the typical Standard American Diet (SAD).

While eating a diet high in good fats, adequate protein, and low in carbohydrates, he only gained three pounds, even though he was consuming 40 percent more calories than his normal daily caloric intake of food.

This illustration above is an example of homeostasis, or energy balance. This occurs when a person is a fat burner on a ketogenic diet, versus being a sugar burner on a high-starch carb diet.

The high-starch carb diet shut down his ability to burn fat because of the constant presence of insulin, the storage hormone. He gained 15 pounds instead of burning the excess calories or eliminating them.

Although he did gain three pounds in the first experiment, he lost an inch and a half around his midsection. In other words, the three pounds he gained was not fat around his middle. **Those three pounds were actually muscle!**

In the second experiment, his waist expanded four inches. No doubt this was due to bloating and water retention, as well as the fat he had accumulated.

Pilgrims, regardless of what you have been told, no one has the intellectual ability to calculate the true calories in and calories out equation.

One simply cannot trust food labels because they are notoriously inaccurate. In addition, there is no accurate way to measure a person's energy output.

However, your body can and will automatically accomplish homeostasis as long as you are hormonally healthy by maintaining a high fat, low carb, moderate protein diet.

Keeping insulin low through carbohydrate restriction is the key to homeostasis.

The real problem with carbohydrates
The real problem with starchy carbohydrates is in the amount of glucose produced by over-ingesting them, which can cause us to develop hyperglycemia, which can be lethal.

However, when too much glucose/sugar is in the bloodstream, the pancreas secretes insulin to remove it, thus eliminating the possibility of hyperglycemia.

Allow me to go into more detail.

Your body follows a **three step process** to remove excess glucose:

1. Insulin is released to unlock certain receptor sites on your cells that allow the glucose to move out of the bloodstream and into our cells for energy production. However, the cells can only use so much glucose at once. When the cells have no need, the excess glucose is left stranded in the blood stream.

2. Insulin is then secreted once again, but this time its job is to carry glucose to the liver, where your body will convert it to glycogen. As you now know, glycogen is another form of sugar, which is stored inside your body for later energy use. However, your muscles and liver can only store a small amount of glycogen. The energy stored in one's liver is used as a backup energy source when our body has no incoming carbohydrates. This is limited to about 100 grams, enough to get us by for three or four hours, depending on activity level. When your glycogen storage areas are full, your body has to come up with a long-term solution to get rid of the excess glucose (from carbohydrates) in your bloodstream.

3. As a last ditch effort, insulin will carry the glucose back to the liver, where the excess glucose is always converted into triglycerides (a type of fat) and then carried (again) by insulin to our cells and pushed into our long-term fat stores.

Excess glucose is stored as FAT! This conversion process is known as lipogenesis.

For men, this is usually around the midsection, back, neck and face. For women, it is typically the thighs, buttocks, and upper arms.

This method of converting excess glucose (from too much carbohydrate consumption) into triglycerides/fat for storage is the way your body stores excess energy for surviving during times of food shortages.

Even though we don't like the effect it has (we become fat), it really is an ingenious mechanism to help with our survival in case of a prolonged food shortage.

The vast majority of people rely primarily on glucose/sugar derived from carbohydrates for fuel. While our bodies can run exclusively on glucose, it's not designed to do so, and the reason is simple. If we are not adapted to burning fat as our primary source of energy we will slowly get fatter over time. This leads to hormonal dysfunction, and can result in heart disease, cancer, Type II Diabetes and Alzheimer's.

Simple and starchy carbohydrates are inherently fattening!

Carbohydrates do not have the satiety factor that protein and fat have, so overeating them is very easy. There is a reason why the advertisers of Lay's potato chips said, "I bet you can't eat just one."

On the other hand, when eating a diet high in fat and moderate in protein, it is nearly impossible to overeat them. A combination of protein and fat fills us up and satisfies our hunger very quickly!

What About Bread?

The bread of our day is not the bread of Jesus' day, Pilgrims.

Our current wheat, barley and rye are actually a low fiber, genetically-modified, nutrient-reduced, and highly-processed product. It also contains gut irritants, of which gluten is the worst. Irritable bowel syndrome and all of its manifestations, including celiac disease, are primarily the result of grains.

Grains also contain excitotoxins, which excite the pleasure centers of the brain. Thus, grains are addictive. They're also the least nutritionally dense of all the food groups. This combination is a recipe for disaster.

In a study published in the Journal of Nutrition in 2007, researchers looked at seven major food groups and 25 subgroups, characterizing the nutrient density of these foods based on the presence of 23 qualifying nutrients (including vitamins, minerals, and protein).

They found that all forms of meat, fish, poultry, nuts, seeds, vegetables, fresh fruits, dairy products, and even legumes were more nutrient-dense than whole grains. In addition, grains wreak havoc on one's digestive system.

The ability to digest food efficiently and eliminate waste products properly is one of the primary keys to optimal health.

About 80 percent of our immune system is contained in our digestive tract. When this system is compromised, we become vulnerable to disease.

When it comes to carbohydrates, all the products from gluten producing grains are unhealthy. Their gut-damaging effects and ability to promote weight gain outweighs what little benefit they may possess.

Therefore, **grains must be avoided** if we are to lose weight/fat and regain optimal digestive health.

Other Carbohydrates

That's not to say all carbs are "bad." Carbohydrates in the form of non-starchy vegetables and low glycemic fruits are far less problematic to our health.

However, starchy vegetables such as potatoes, rice, and corn are sticky. By that, I mean they will stick to your ribs, and they must be avoided **until** you are lean! Your consumption of carbohydrates on this eating plan will be limited to a safe quantity of high quality carbs that will not predispose you to metabolic dysfunction.

When it comes to the subject of starches, some will tell you there are some safe starches, such as white potatoes and white rice, which you may consume.

The previous statement is only true in the context of anyone who has depleted their liver and muscle glycogen after **intense exercise over a long period.**

Think in terms of a three-hour football game, two-hour intense basketball game, or after an eight-hour day of hard physical work!

As Dr. John Berardi says, you should "earn your starches".

In that way, the consumed starch will be used immediately for energy, and the excess, if any, will be converted to glycogen and stored in the liver and skeletal muscle for later use.

In other words, you have to work hard for your starches FIRST. Then, eat them ONLY AFTER you are glycogen depleted, or else those starches will end up as fat.

I used to eat a baked potato every day, and I weighed 253 pounds!

Now that I have regained my health AND reached my ideal weight, I will eat a baked potato occasionally only if I have played basketball for a couple of hours that day!

The key here is (1) I am already at my target weight, and (2) I earned my starches (carbohydrates) with strenuous physical activity BEFORE I ate them!

On the other hand, **non-starchy vegetables** will not cause weight gain, so enjoy all of them that you want, within reason. These include broccoli, cauliflower, lettuce, spinach, and many other delicious non-starchy vegetables.

These non-starchy vegetables are a powerhouse of vitamins, minerals, and antioxidants. Gram for gram, they contain eight times more fiber than grain, as well as nature's purified water via osmosis.

I have learned to love them and enjoy them every day.

Beans, Beans, The Musical Fruit…

Please note that beans are 60-80 percent starch, and also contain a sugar (oligosaccharides) humans cannot digest. The result usually includes all manner of unpleasant digestive issues and embarrassing moments.

For **now,** bounce the beans back in the barrel and leave them there, Pilgrims.

Fruit

Once you become lean and reach your ideal bodyweight, fruit is fine in small quantities. Always remember, fruit is part of a healthy diet for those who are already healthy and lean. Fructose, the specific type of sugar found in fruit, is very burdensome to the liver and is perceived by our bodies as toxic, because no cell in our body can directly utilize fructose!

Every gram of fructose we consume must go through the detox organ, the liver, where it can be converted into glycogen if needed. If it isn't needed, it will be converted into fat/triglycerides and stored, primarily in the liver, where it becomes the major cause of non-alcoholic fatty liver disease.

Fructose corn syrup is as damaging to the liver as alcohol is to an alcoholic. In healthy people, fruit is not an issue if eaten in small quantities of one or two servings per day. Low glycemic fruit choices like those in the berry family are the best. Their fiber, vitamins, and minerals plus antioxidants are part of a healthy diet for healthy people and will not spike insulin, because it does not raise blood glucose.

The Danger Of 'Simple' Carbs (Sugary Drinks)

Of all carbs, simple carbohydrates are the most fattening and damaging to your health. To add insult to injury, they're highly addictive.

Soda drinks are full of high fructose corn syrup, perhaps the number one factor contributing to rising obesity in America. A can of soda pop contains 12-16 teaspoons of sugar. No one in their right mind would consume that much table sugar, but few think twice about consuming two or three cans of pop a day!

We must be wise in the choices that we make concerning what type of carbohydrates we will eat. If we are, they will serve us well. If we are not, they will be our undoing!

Sugar

On the Pilgrim's Plan, you will consume very little sugar. Ideally, none will come from processed foods like candy, cookies, cake, ice cream or soda pop.

Sugar is highly addictive and triggers the same pleasure centers in the brain as cocaine!

The massive overconsumption of sugar, plus chemically-laced processed food, is a leading cause of cancer, cardiovascular disease, dementia, obesity, and Type II Diabetes.

When sugar was scarce and processed foods were not available, virtually none of the modern diseases existed.

Today, the average American consumes more sugar in a day than their grandparents did in a week, more in a week than their great grandparents did in a month, and more in a month than their great great grandparents did in a year, and more in a year than their great-great great grandparents did in a lifetime!

We have become sugar addicts.

The average American consumes more than 152 pounds of sugar a year. Compare that to about ten pounds per year in the early 1800s.

That's just the average. When one considers that many people consume more than the average, it is no wonder obesity and Type II Diabetes is a pandemic in America.

Sugar is extremely addictive and kills more people every year than all illegal drugs combined. It also kills three times more people than cigarettes annually.

If the good Lord delays his return for another 50 years, that future generation will look back and be dumbfounded at our sugar addiction.

 Unfortunately, they will be in the same boat and heading over the falls unless you and I throw them a lifeline! The Pilgrim's Plan is that lifeline!

Up to this point, I have been referring to the sugar we add to coffee or tea, or foods baked at home. This includes the sweeteners that food manufacturers add to processed food and drinks.

High fructose corn syrup, trans fats, and all the chemical additives in processed foods, are the most damaging to our health.

The chemicals are, no doubt, the root cause of the ever-increasing cancer rates, and high fructose corn syrup is the main culprit driving non-alcoholic fatty liver disease, Type II Diabetes, and obesity.

Critical Point:
All carbohydrates are converted
into sugar/glucose by your liver.

All carbohydrates, simple or complex, are converted to sugar when consumed. This type of sugar is called glucose and every cell in your body can use it for energy.

However, EXCESS carbohydrates are always converted into triglycerides/fat and stored in our adipose (fat) deposit.

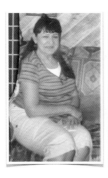 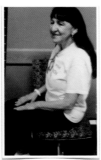

Lynn Todd: 60 Pounds Lost! These pictures show me at close to 200 lbs, size 16 then, and 140 pounds, size 10 now!

Not too many weeks went by until I asked Patty about this life change for her and Dennis. She shared 'The Pilgrim's Plan' with me. So I followed the plan.

Within 10-14 days my clothes started feeling loose. That gave me encouragement to continue. That was in 2012. I have been size 10 and 140 pounds for over 2 years now!

Lynn Todd

SECTION THREE:

LEVERAGING REAL FOOD

FOR NATURAL FAT LOSS

CHAPTER SIX

WE ARE HYBRIDS

"I praise you because of the wonderful way you created me"
(Psalm 139:14, CEV).

Pilgrims, our bodies are amazing! David said, "I praise you because of the wonderful way you created me" (Psalm 139:14, CEV). I completely agree with him! After watching how my body responded to a change in diet and the almost immediate surge of energy and vitality I experienced, I am more aware than ever of our body's natural ability to heal itself, if given the proper nutrients.

One important fact about our bodies that most people don't know is that we actually have two energy systems inside our body. In fact, we are somewhat like the Toyota Prius, which also has two power sources. It can run on gasoline or electricity.

Most people use carbohydrates/glucose exclusively for energy. However, we can convert our bodies to use the more efficient fuel, ketones, for energy!

We typically classify these two states as being a sugar burner or a fat burner.

Sugar Burners
Sugar burners have about 400 calories of energy which to draw from before they must eat again, otherwise they will experience the infamous carb crash or what athletes call hitting the wall. The person adapted to burning fat

for fuel has infinitely more energy available than a sugar burner has, and never crashes! If you are a sugar burner only, you will have to refuel every three to four hours. This makes you a slave to food and the clock on the wall. When you are about to run out of fuel, food is always on your mind.

Fat Burners
In ketosis we always burn a combination of both fat and glucose simultaneously, but the predominant energy source is fat.

Certain parts of our body do require glucose for operation.

For example, a portion of our brain, one-fourth, must have glucose.

However, the other three-fourths of our brain operates optimally and very efficiently on ketones.

Our hearts prefer ketones for fuel, but like the brain, the heart can run exclusively on glucose if required to do so.

One other interesting note is that our red-blood cells must have glucose exclusively, as well as the retina of our eyes and a portion (the medulla) of the kidney.

With a few exceptions, the body, as a whole, prefers ketones to glucose. It is a slow, clean-burning energy source, which promotes longevity of life, and your body has a vast supply of it. Let's look at some examples.

You've probably already heard that a pound of fat represents 3,500 calories that have been stored on your body. Essentially, this represents stored energy, which is available to use when our body needs it. This is only true if one's body can access it.

Let's assume we have a 160-pound man with 10 percent body fat. This means he has approximately 16 pounds of fat in reserve, which will supply 56,000 units of caloric energy at his disposal if he has adapted his body to burning fat.

This same man with 20 percent body fat would have 112,000 caloric units of energy to use.

Once you have become adapted to using fat as your energy source, you can easily go 16-18 hours between your last meal of the day, until your first meal the next day with no drop in energy.

Why? Because your body will metabolize the fat in your body, as needed, to get the energy that it needs.

This is a real game-changer!

This is possible because of the vast energy source that is available in your fat stores.

When In Ketosis, You Have An Extra Fuel Tank!
Take a close look at this fuel tank on the next page.

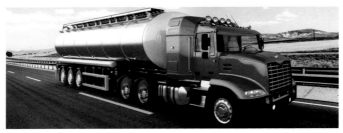

The small, silver, fuel tanks on the side of the tractor represent all the fuel he has available to use. Yet he is carrying a vast amount of fuel.

Now, imagine if he could open up a valve and tap into that huge tanker full of fuel.

That is YOU in the state of ketosis!

A sugar-burner has about 400 calories of energy to draw from until they must eat again, and yet the average person has about 100,000 calories stored in body fat. **That is over two hundred fifty times more energy that is available to you than a sugar-burner has available.**

This fuel is a cleaner, efficient, slow burning fuel that causes less wear and tear on your body.

Twigs Or Logs?
Let's look at another example.

Imagine you live in a cabin and heat it with a wood stove. All you have for fuel is newspaper, kindling, some twigs, and lighter fluid.

You fill up your fireplace with the kindling and twigs you found, douse a little lighter fluid on the newspaper, and light a match. Presto! You have made a fire and a very hot one. In fifteen minutes, the fire goes out, and you scramble frantically picking up small sticks and twigs to repeat the process. Sure enough, fifteen minutes later, you go scrambling again for more kindling. You are a slave to that stove. It's on your mind constantly.

Instead of fueling your fire with twigs and kindling that burn fast and hot, you could use a big log in that stove, a log that would burn for hours. This strategic change would be far less stressful, and certainly more efficient.

What a liberating moment that would be!

Pilgrims, I think you can see where I'm going with this example!

Just switch from twigs/glucose as your primary energy source to logs/ketones, and you'll live a lot longer with a whole lot less stress!

So What Does This Mean?
By now, you are probably realizing that your body can produce fuel in two ways, both through carbohydrate/glucose metabolism, and also through ketone bodies produced from your vast reservoir of stored fat.

Glucose burns fast and hot leaving a lot of gunk, free radicals, after the burn! These free radicals are what ages us as the body fights hard to get rid of them.

The good news is that when you are a fat/ketone burner, you get the best of both worlds. You still have glycogen in your muscles to use in fight-or-flight situations, AND you also have a vast clean-energy source. Your body can access and burn fat efficiently through the miracle of becoming a fat-burner.

The research is clear on this point. "We know muscles still store glycogen in ketosis, as this has been well studied," Dr. Peter Attia.

What I just described is your most optimal state. Your body is burning ketones/fat for your primary energy source, and then uses the stored glycogen in your muscles for the short, quick bursts of energy you need in emergencies or when playing sports.

Two Energy Systems

As we mentioned above, your body actually has **TWO** energy systems! Everyone needs to know how this works.

Carbohydrates will break down into glucose, which can be used for energy. You should be keenly aware that fat can also be used by your body to create energy to fuel life. Not many people know this, yet it is a scientific fact.

The truth is that you have two complementary energy systems in your body. One energy system burns sugar/glucose, and the other burns fat/ketones.

When a person is dependent on burning sugar/glucose for energy, this state of energy metabolism is called being a **"sugar burner."**

While you are carrying around excess fat stores I can guarantee your body is in "sugar burning" mode rather than "fat burning" mode. Making matters worse is that you cannot access your fat stores for energy. Thus, you must eat every few hours to guarantee a steady flow of vital energy! You are trapped in a "must eat" mode every three or four hours.

This explains the "late night snack" syndrome. This late night snack prevents a sugar-burner from experiencing low blood sugar, also called hypoglycemia, which causes one to feel shaky, nervous, hungry and confused.

We have all experienced the roller coaster ride of a high carb meal. At first we feel great from our high! Soon we begin to feel sluggish, tired, and weak. We need a nap. Some people eat a light lunch to avoid this problem. After all, they need to be productive for the rest of the day. Falling asleep at one's desk certainly isn't productive.

At their mid-afternoon break, they load up on caffeine and a sugary snack in order to complete their workday, which is not a healthy scenario.

These are just a few of the issues a person must deal with when our body is dependent on glucose/sugar exclusively for its energy demands.

I want to re-emphasize a VERY important point:

All carbs are converted to sugar/glucose, and yes, the brain must have **some** sugar/glucose to fuel its activities.

However, your liver can produce enough glucose daily to keep the brain healthy **without ingesting any carbs!**

The brain only requires approximately 130 grams of glucose

per day when using it for its primary energy source. However, it can run on 75 percent ketones, a by-product of fat metabolism, and function more efficiently than on glucose!

It is a scientific fact that our bodies have no dependence on ingested carbohydrates.

We can produce all the glucose we need from protein or fat and create the small amount of glucose needed for the brain.

My point is three-fold:

1. Carbs are non-essential to sustain life according to the USDA.

2. Your liver can produce all the glucose it needs to sustain life from ingested protein or fat through gluconeogenesis.

3. Starchy-carb consumption results in weight gain, **unless** consumed after intense exercise, when glycogen stores have been depleted.

Following this logic leads us to this MAJOR point:

Starchy carbohydrates will make you FAT unless you carefully control the timing of their consumption to only post-workout recovery or after a hard day of manual labor.

Eating fat does not make you fat!
It is almost impossible to get fat by eating fat, **unless the**

fat is consumed with starchy carbohydrates or sugar laden desserts, drinks, etc.. This is true because the satiety factor of fat makes it unlikely anyone would overeat it. Simply put, you feel full when you eat healthy fat and don't want to overeat.

By comparison, when eating carbohydrates (the least satiating of the three macronutrients), you never feel full. This causes a dangerous cycle of overconsumption of carbs. This causes your insulin levels to rise, which prevents the burning of fat.

The Pilgrim's Plan of eating is low carb, has adequate protein, and is high in "good fats." My plan will ensure you lose fat without calorie restriction or hunger.

The key to avoiding fat accumulation is starchy carbohydrate restriction, which keeps insulin levels low. Your fat storage mechanisms never get activated!

> "When insulin is low, fat will go.
> When insulin is high, fat will rise."
> Ken Burge

When you are in ketosis, eating a high fat diet does not make you fat. Instead, it enhances your fat-burning capabilities.

Once you have reached your ideal weight, you stop losing weight by just eating more, high-quality carbohydrates. This is where you would add back into your diet starchy vegetables, like sweet potatoes or beans if you can tolerate them. If the scale starts creeping upward, just back the carbs down a wee bit.

Remember, fat cells never completely go away. They can

shrink in size or they can blow up like a balloon in an incredibly short time, depending on your hormonal balance.

Nothing is harder on your body than yo-yoing up and down the scale. For optimal health, remaining within a few pounds of your ideal weight is critical.

Pilgrims, do not fear the fat!

Not only does eating fat not make you fat, you must eat a high-fat diet in order to lose fat.

Sounds crazy, right? I assure you, it's not.

Once I got over my disbelief and put into practice the principles outlined in this book, I lost 80 pounds of fat in just a few months.

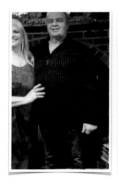 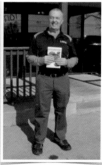

Phil Jackson: 49 Pounds Lost!
I am in my 50's and have fought controlling my weight all of my life.

This way of eating gives you energy every day, does not leave you hungry, will absolutely control your weight and makes your mind more alert.

I lost 49 pounds and I did this with no exercise program involved to get there! What have you got to lose?

Phil Jackson

CHAPTER SEVEN

HOW TO EAT FOR OPTIMAL HEALTH AND HEALING

"Dear friend, I pray that you may enjoy
good health and that all may go well with you,
even as your soul is getting along well"
(3 John 2, NIV).

The Pilgrim's Plan for Optimal Health is a way of eating that is both enjoyable and sustainable for the rest of your life. My meals are super delicious, highly nutritious and very filling. I never leave the table wishing I could eat just a little more or afraid to do so!

I want to stress this fact to you, my friends; I lost 80 pounds of ugly fat eating this way, and gained enormous amounts of energy!

We all know people who lost weight on a fad diet and then promptly regained the weight, or even more.

Why? There are two reasons:

1. Their diet was calorie restricted, as in a starvation diet that could not be sustained long term.

2. They were allowed to continue eating the same things that caused their weight gain in the first place, just a lot less of them! Therefore, this did not fix their hormonal imbalance, and therefore, the weight was destined to return when they gave up on the starvation diet.

Once these people increased the amount of food they were eating, they naturally started the whole cycle again, gaining even more weight than when they began their diet.

Pilgrims I am very pleased to tell you that…

I HAVE MAINTAINED MY FAT LOSS EFFORT-LESSLY FOR OVER SIX YEARS! PRAISE THE LORD!

When you follow the recommendations in this book, you will naturally consume a high fat, adequate protein and low carb diet.

This way of eating has a long track record of producing lean, healthy, disease-free people.

There is no need to count calories on this plan, because **this is not a calorie-restricted diet.** Willpower is not a factor when eating this way, because you need never be hungry or feel deprived. **Always eat when hungry, but only when hungry.** Don't be a slave to the clock or someone else's schedule.

You won't need to refuel every three or four hours on this eating plan, because you will have a constant, steady flow of energy coming from stored body fat. This becomes your primary energy source.

You will easily be able to go 16 hours or longer between your evening meal and your first meal the next day. This allows time for your digestive system to thoroughly do its work before the next meal arrives.

Problematic Foods

The first phase of this plan is to eliminate food groups that are problematic for most people to digest. This phase will also detox your body from the toxins contained in processed foods!

If you cannot properly digest and assimilate the nutrients in the food you eat, one of two things will happen. You will end up with malnutrition, and/or you will set yourself up for disease.

For example, many people are lactose intolerant and cannot digest the sugar in milk. I suffered from a "dis-ease" called diarrhea for years, before I figured out what my problem was.

We also know that it is gluten in wheat, barley and rye that causes celiac disease. Irritable bowel syndrome, Crohn's, leaky gut, bloating, and more have all been linked to grain products.

Legumes and beans contain gut irritants and sugars humans cannot digest. The latter results in excessive gas and very embarrassing moments when in public. Beans also have a high starch content, which leads to weight gain.

Eat Real Food

It is vitally important that the food we eat is recognized by our body as real food. Our bodies simply will not operate well on man-made foods, which are full of toxic chemicals, preservatives, food coloring, and MSG.

If we want to be healthy, we must eat natural, nutrient-dense foods.

So just what is real food?

Well Pilgrims, if it grows out of the ground or it has a mother, it's real food! This definition also includes the natural occurring minerals and vitamins that our body requires, which we typically get through the real food we consume.

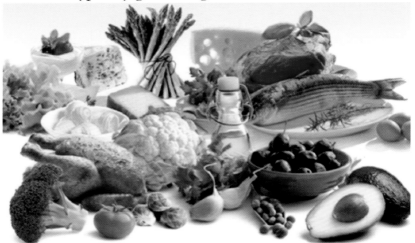

When it comes to the healing of our bodies, nothing is as powerful and effective as real food.

God, in his infinite wisdom, created the body with the amazing ability to heal itself, when given the proper food to do so. "Let food be thy medicine - thy medicine thy food" (Hippocrates, 460-377 BC).

The Pilgrim's way of eating boils down to this: Avoid highly processed Frankenfood loaded with sugar, salt, and disease-producing chemicals. Plus, eliminate foods that cause you gastrointestinal stress!

Eat real, natural food, which is low in starchy carbohydrates, moderate in protein, and high in the good, healthy fats. This will keep your insulin levels low so that your body can easily access and burn your fat stores.

Simply put, being overweight is the result of not being able to access your fat stores for energy.

As you read this book, you are learning how to tap into your fat stores and burn the excess fat away.

The Pilgrim's Plan is sustainable and enjoyable for the rest of your life. Once again, consider the incredible benefits you will enjoy!

Nine Incredible Benefits of Becoming A Fat Burner

1. Effortless weight loss, especially belly fat, as your body learns to burn fat.

2. No more Carb-Coma — this plan eliminates the roller-coaster ride by design.

3. You'll experience a dramatic increase in energy with a steady release all day long.

4. Naturally lowers your blood sugar, thereby preventing Type II Diabetes.

5. Naturally lowers your blood pressure, guarding against stroke and heart attack.

6. Naturally lowers your triglycerides, the major indicator of cardiovascular disease.

7. Good cholesterol (HDL) will increase...vital for proper hormonal balance.

8. Your mental clarity will vastly improve. Brain fog will go away and memory will greatly improve.

9. No more digestive issues such as bloating, heartburn, constipation, or diarrhea!

So, What Do We Eat On This Plan?

The obvious question at this point is, "So…what can we eat on the Pilgrim's Plan?" I've included a brief overview below. These nine broad categories offer tremendous variety and will bring many health benefits to you.

Nine Everyday Essential Real Foods

1. Beef

The word protein is derived from a Greek word meaning, "of first importance." Without this essential macronutrient, we would die. Our muscles are made, maintained, and repaired by consuming protein. **Red meat is health food, when consumed in moderate quantities.** Study after study has debunked the myth that red meat causes cancer, or that its saturated fat causes cardiovascular disease. Just don't overeat protein. Any amount over your daily requirement to build, maintain, or repair muscle tissue will be converted to glucose by the liver and stored as fat. Protein is never wasted by the body, it cannot be stored as protein, but it can, however, be converted to fat, which obviously can be stored.

**Important Note:
The Pilgrim's Plan is NOT a high protein diet!**

On the other hand, if you don't consume adequate amounts of protein, you will lose muscle mass. I recommend a portion the size of the palm of your hand at each meal, and consume two portions if your work is physically demanding. Try this recommendation for a month and then adjust according to your specific needs.

Beef that has been fed only grass and no grains, is best, but not necessary for this plan to work for you.

2. Fowl

Chicken or turkey is excellent protein. Be sure to eat the skin, because the fat is good for you. In fact, it will help you LOSE fat. I cannot over-stress the importance of consuming high quality fats in your pursuit of becoming a fat burner.

3. Pork

My favorite is barbecued ribs with no sauce! How about some pork chops or a good smoked ham? Pilgrims, I can't imagine a day without bacon.

4. Fish

Salmon, trout, sardines, and other fish are excellent sources of protein. Each contains the essential fatty acid omega 3, which is excellent for your brain. The old saying that fish is brain food is correct.

5. Eggs

The incredible, edible egg is perhaps the most perfect food. It is a nutritional powerhouse and ideal for a ketogenic diet, although it has been demonized unfairly for the past 40 years. Now the truth is coming out that the humble egg is not the enemy to your health that it has been accused of being.

Just look at this Time magazine cover shown on the next page.

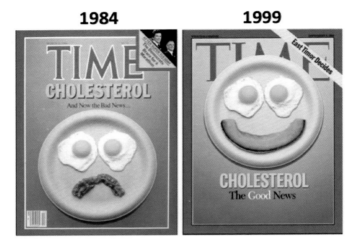

The egg yolk is the best part and full of essential nutrients. Two to three eggs per meal is about right for most people. Eggs are easily digested and high in omega 3 essential fatty acids. Free-range hen eggs are the best tasting and the best for you. When it's possible, always buy organic eggs.

6. Vegetables (non-starchy only)

Non-starchy vegetables are full of vitamins, minerals, and antioxidants essential to good health. They are low in calories and high in fiber, plus their water content has been purified by nature through the process of osmosis. I recommend two or three cups per day minimum! When eating vegetables, always use liberal quantities of olive oil or full fat, sugar-free salad dressings or real butter. I always dip my broccoli and cauliflower in melted butter.

7. Fruit

Caution: I recommend one or two servings per day, but only after you have reached your ideal weight and have regained your health. Berries are the best choice.

They contain less fructose/sugar and have more fiber, as well as more vitamins, minerals, and antioxidants than most other fruit choices.

8. Nuts and seeds

A handful of Macadamia nuts, which are lightly salted with sea salt, are my favorite. I also enjoy pecans, walnuts, pumpkin seeds, and sunflower seeds.

9. Collagen Peptide Protein Powder (CPP)

Collagen peptide protein powder and zero carb isolate protein are my two exceptions when it comes to avoiding processed foods. In addition, this supplement does wonders for your skin, hair, nails, and helps your joints and ligaments as well! I use Collagen Peptides from Sports Research.

This product mixes very well in hot or cold beverages such as coffee or tea. It is also an excellent addition to a smoothie or post-workout protein shake!

These nine food categories are delicious and nutritious. There are dozens of ways to mix and match to make them interesting and savory.

Remember to use healthy animal fats or coconut oil for cooking to add flavor to your recipes. But, never use vegetable oils, which increase inflation.

Eating high-quality, natural-healthy fats plays a major role in becoming a fat burner. This is the fastest way to reach your ideal weight and regain your health.

Foods To Avoid At All Costs

Just as there are items you must add to your diet to become

a fat burner, there are also items that you must eliminate in order for your body to get the proper hormonal signals that it is ok to access your fat stores and burn them for energy. Let me share with you the nine items you MUST remove from your diet to become a fat burner:

Nine Foods You Must Eliminate From Your Diet For Now

1. Eliminate starchy vegetables for now.

Consume low calorie, high fiber, and non-starchy vegetables to your heart's content. No one ever got fat eating this class of carbohydrate!

2. Eliminate all grains.

Farmers feed grain to cattle to fatten them up for market. The so-called beer belly is actually a grain belly. Therefore, go against the grain. Grains are the least nutrient-dense food groups, and it is the gluten in wheat, barley, and rye that is responsible for bloating, excess gas, and digestive disorders such as celiac, Crohn's disease, and irritable bowel syndrome. Grains are also addictive, and they trigger the pleasure centers in the brain, making it harder to wean oneself away from them. Dr. William Davis MD says, "…to food manufacturers, wheat is like nicotine in cigarettes and is the best insurance they have to encourage continued consumption." Don't think you must eat grains in order to get enough fiber in your diet. You will get all the fiber required for regularity and optimal colon health by eating non-starchy vegetables.

3. Eliminate all dairy products for now

Two exceptions are butter and heavy cream that have the lactose/sugar and problematic casein protein removed. Butter and cream are fat, and fat is your best friend in the pursuit of reaching a fat-adapted state. Milk is the perfect food for baby calves, but they are soon weaned and turned to grass for their nutrition. Breast milk is the perfect food for our babies as well, but only for a short time until they are able to digest solid food. Most adults find themselves unable to digest the lactose/sugar in milk. The result of this is not pretty or comfortable. If you have no intolerance issue with dairy, then congratulations to you! If you have access to raw, unpasteurized, full-fat milk products from a local dairy farm with grass-fed cows, go ahead and enjoy. You are kidding yourself if you think your local grocery store is providing a healthy dairy product.

4. Eliminate all legumes/beans for now

Beans are extremely high in starchy carbohydrates (60-80 percent) and very low in fat. It is no wonder that those who make beans the staple of their diet are generally overweight. Beans also contain a sugar called oligosaccharide, which humans cannot digest. The result is methane gas, as well as a great deal of discomfort, not to mention embarrassment. (Note: green beans are the exception to this rule).

5. Eliminate fruit for now

The sugar/fructose in fruit is the problem. It is partially responsible for Non-Alcoholic Fatty Liver Disease (NAFLD), which is life threatening. Here is why.

No cell in the body can use fructose, so it is perceived as a toxin.

In order for your body to assimilate fructose, it is sent to our detox organ, the liver, which then converts the fructose into triglycerides/fat. Unfortunately, most of it accumulates in and around the liver and contributes to NAFLD.

This visceral fat, or fat accumulation around internal organs, is the most dangerous and the most difficult to eradicate. Eliminating fruit from your diet while you are trying to lose weight is the right thing to do.

In case you are thinking that I have gone too far in suggesting that you eliminate fruit, remember I said for now. **Once you reach your ideal weight, you may have fruit in small quantities.** The berry family is your best choice because they contain less fructose, more fiber, vitamins, minerals, and antioxidants than most other fruit.

6. Eliminate all processed foods

This is basically anything that comes in a can or box with a label containing un-pronounceable words. Generally speaking, that includes everything in the middle aisles of the grocery store.

Pilgrims, processed 'foods' make up 80 percent of the 'food' in our stores today!

These manufactured foods are chock full of toxic chemicals, as well as sugar and salt!

Your transition to eating real food will be much easier than you may think. The new foods you will be consuming will take away your hunger cravings for these addictive foods and give you far more energy than you have today.

7. Say goodbye to all fast-food establishments

If you have no other choice, just order a salad with

grilled chicken. Be sure to ask for full-fat dressing. If salad is not your thing, order a cheeseburger without the bun and omit the fries. Ask for water to drink. The key to staying on track when eating out is to take charge of the situation. Decide right now what your course of action will be. You can always order some sort of meat and a vegetable, if you are caught in this situation. Resolve to minimize your visits to these establishments.

8. Eliminate all vegetable oils

They are very high in omega 6, which increases inflammation and drives every modern-day disease. They also may contain hydrogenated trans fats, which may be one of the leading causes of cancer. Cook with butter, bacon drippings, beef tallow, coconut oil, lard, and olive oil. These are not only healthy for you, but they also add great flavor. Plus, because they are fat, they help you get even more of the good, healthy fat into your diet, which is necessary to becoming a fat burner.

9. Eliminate all sugar for now

I am sure that you noticed the words **"for now"** a lot in this chapter. After you have reached your ideal weight and regained your health, you may slowly reintroduce these **"for now"** foods back into your diet.

I emphasize that you do this slowly with one food group at a time. Monitor how your body responds. If you experience nausea, bloating, excess gas, cramping, diarrhea, or constipation, then you should permanently eliminate that food group.

Pilgrims, your body grumbles when it is trying to tell you something. Be wise and listen to your body. However, I am not suggesting adding table sugar (sucrose) back into your diet once your goal has been achieved.

If you must have some sweetener in your coffee or tea, use a little natural stevia. **Once you have regained your health,** small quantities of low glycemic fruit, organic if possible, and local honey may become a small part of your diet. **Small quantities of dark chocolate are allowed too! Praise The Lord.**

Salt

The amount of salt you use daily to give more flavor to your food will not raise your blood pressure. Salt is an essential mineral electrolyte and doesn't cause high blood pressure, yet we've been told this myth for a long time.

The grossly excessive amount of salt in processed food could create an imbalance with potassium, resulting in hypertension in people who are predisposed to high blood pressure.

The real cause of hypertension is insulin resistance, due to a high processed carbohydrate diet. Therefore, since you will be eating very little, if any, processed food on the plan outlined in this book, I encourage you to continue using your saltshaker.

However, please upgrade from common table salt to a high quality sea salt. It contains essential trace minerals, which promote good health. Pink Himalayan is my favorite.

During the elimination phase of this plan, your digestion will greatly improve and your blood sugar and blood pressure will improve as well.

Be sure to keep hydrated and don't forget to make sure you are consuming adequate amounts of essential electrolytes: salt, potassium, and magnesium. This will prevent any light-headedness, constipation, or muscle-cramping, which could occur while making this transition from being a sugar burner to a fat burner.

Summary

This part of the Pilgrim's Plan is about eating real, unprocessed food and eliminating food groups that are known to wreak havoc on proper digestion and elimination processes.

Switching to real foods will cause you to experience weight loss. For some people, it may be significant. However, the primary benefit will be much-improved digestion, better nutrient absorption from the real foods you are eating, and a reduction in hunger cravings.

In the next few chapters, I'm going to share with you the secret of putting your fat loss into high gear. You will start to enter into nutritional dietary ketosis and your body will naturally and easily be able to efficiently burn your stored fat for fuel.

But first, let me illustrate a typical day in my life.

CHAPTER EIGHT

A DAY IN THE LIFE...

"This is the day that the Lord has made;
we will rejoice and be glad in it"
(Psalm 118:24, NKJV).

Let me walk you through a typical day in my life and, step by step, illustrate how I apply the information I have shared. First, we'll look at what I eat.

Remember, this is how I eat since I have reached my ideal weight. During the period when I wanted to burn off more fat, I modified this routine to exclude any fruit.

A Day In The Life of the Pilgrim

My day starts at 6 a.m. with two cups of cold water while my strong coffee is brewing. Drinking chilled water can give the metabolism a morning boost. I take an omega three supplement and vitamin D3. I put one tablespoon of MCT oil and one tablespoon of butter in my coffee. I have another cup at 9 a.m. This is a great way to start the day with healthy fats that help you train your body to burn fat for fuel.

At noon, I have two options. I either eat three large eggs, three thick slices of bacon, and an avocado, or I make a protein replacement meal in the form of a shake.

I make this shake with one scoop of collagen peptide protein powder and or, according to your needs, one scoop of zero carb protein isolate, one avocado, one cup of frozen strawberries, a little Stevia to sweeten things, ice cubes, and water. Remember, I include strawberries (fruit) in my shake because I have already reached my goal weight. **During your fat loss phase, you will want to eliminate all fruit from this shake.**

This makes a very thick shake that is smooth like pudding, delicious, and very nutritious meal replacement. This is very filling and normally keeps me satisfied until my evening meal on the days I choose to have a shake instead of a full conventional meal.

In the late afternoon, **if I am hungry,** I will eat a handful of macadamia nuts! **Pilgrims, never eat if you are not hungry!** Always let your appetite and not your emotions or a clock dictate when you eat.

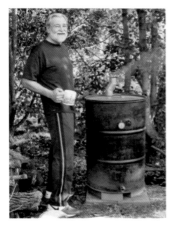

At 6 p.m., I eat two or three cups of non-starchy vegetables. Broccoli, dipped in melted butter, is my favorite, and a half-dozen green olives, and an avocado.

I also will eat a portion or two of beef, chicken, pork, or fish the size of the palm of my hand.

Now that I have completely regained my health, I will, on occasion, have a cup of berries with heavy cream for dessert.

It is at this time I also take an enzyme supplement, to help me break down the fat I have consumed and better digest my food. I also take a Turmeric/Curcumin supplement at this time. Turmeric helps control blood sugar and removes plaque that can lead to Alzheimer's. It also reduces inflammation and helps prevent cancer!

Let's talk about water.

It's going to be critical to your success, as it will help you avoid dehydration and helps with satiety (feeling of fullness).

However, you may be surprised to know that I drink very little water with my meals. This prevents my digestive juices from being diluted while eating and ensures proper digestion.

However, throughout the day, I drink plenty of water as we all should. Ultimately, you want to always let your thirst guide you, as long as you know how to listen for the signals of thirst.

One way to check to see if you are getting enough water is to look to see if your urine is always clear and never dark. Dark urine is a clear indication to drink more water!

As a general rule, this is how I calculate how much water to drink each day:

Take your bodyweight and divide by 2. This number will be the number of ounces of water you should drink each day.

For example: 160 lbs of bodyweight ÷ 2 = 80 ounces

In this example, this 160 lb person should try to drink at least 80 ounces of water per day. I encourage you to drink most of this before 4 p.m. in the afternoon so that you don't go to bed with a full bladder, which could interrupt your sleep.

Meal Planning: K.I.S.S (Keep It Super Simple)

I highly recommend that you adopt the philosophy that the above acronym suggests. Keep it super simple! What I'm talking about here is meal planning. For now, just follow the guidelines that I have provided for you, rather than trying to over-complicate things. When you follow the guidelines in this book, your body will have no choice but to enter into nutritional ketosis and burn fat naturally.

So, how should you put together a healthy meal?

Choose a good quality protein source you really enjoy and a non-starchy vegetable as well. (see Appendix B)

Mix these two items together **making sure** to add an adequate amount of a high quality fat source to satisfy your hunger. Avocados, olives, and nuts are the easiest and healthiest way to add a high quality fat, so that you satisfy your hunger (satiety).

Just simply rotate these meals until you have reached your goal!

Important Note:

To stay in ketosis, you must stay under 50 grams of carbohydrates daily. Your daily protein grams are determined by your weight, age, gender, and activity level and won't vary much day to day. That leaves fat as the variable quantity from day to day, based on your hunger level.

Now back to my daily schedule…

I read from 7 p.m. to 9 p.m. and spend quality time with my wife. We also pray for one another and our family. Then we share our day's activities and plan our tomorrow.

From 9 p.m. to 10 p.m., I practice quiet prayer and meditation in preparation for an energizing great night of sleep.

It is at this time that I take a supplement called ZMA, which contributes to a good night's rest. The brand I use is called 'Now'.

You may have noticed I eat within a six-hour period of time. This means I am practicing intermittent fasting 18 hours every day. You'll learn more about this in upcoming chapters, but this is a scientifically proven strategy for fat loss and longevity of life.

How am I able to do this and yet have such an abundance of energy throughout the whole day?

The key is the MCT oil and butter that I consume each morning with my coffee and the high quality fats I eat from noon to 6 pm.

I am in ketosis burning fat for energy 24/7 and never lack for energy!

I never go hungry and I never restrict calories. It certainly helps that I love bacon and eggs any time of day. However, I suggest you mix and match from the approved foods on this plan and create a satisfying combination for your palate. These foods are delicious, nutritious, and satiating!

Let's do a quick review of what a plate should look like in order for you to receive all the vitamins, minerals, antioxidants, and essential fatty acids that are necessary to experience optimal health. You will lose fat and never go hungry.

1. A portion or two, depending upon your needs, of high quality protein the size of the palm of your hand.

2. At least two or three cups of non-starchy vegetables with butter or extra virgin olive oil.

3. A plate should have enough of a healthy fat source—avocado is my favorite—to satiate your hunger. The avocado also ensures you are getting enough, soluble fiber in your diet to go with the insoluble fiber from the veggies.

Pilgrims, I have a confession to make. I love chocolate! I eat several small pieces of Green & Black's 85 percent organic dark chocolate **almost** every day! Believe me, the benefits of dark chocolate outweigh the liabilities!

There are multiple studies showing dark chocolate has powerful health benefits, including improved blood flow, lower blood pressure, and improved brain function. One study stated that consuming dark chocolate five times per week lowered the risk of heart disease by 57 percent. It contains more antioxidants than blueberries!

Let's be honest, Pilgrims, my plan is not all that tough, is it?

I eat bacon, eggs, nuts, seeds, avocados, and a little chocolate. I also enjoy steak, ribs, pork chops, chicken, hamburger, heavy cream, and lots of butter. I also eat plenty of green veggies, such as broccoli, spinach, and green beans.

Anybody can do this! **We did!**

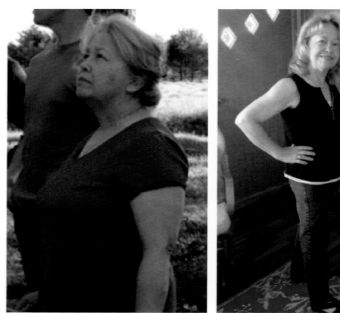

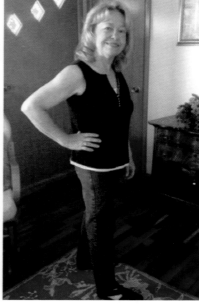

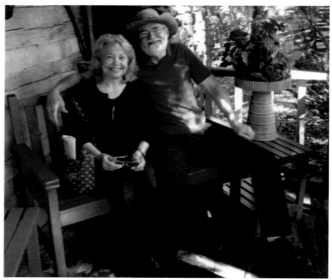

SECTION FOUR:

TURBOCHARGING YOUR FAT LOSS

CHAPTER NINE

TURBOCHARGED FAT LOSS WITH KETOSIS

"I will give you the best of the land of Egypt,
and you will eat the fat of the land"
(Genesis 45:18, NKJV).

I want to introduce to you a natural way to turbocharge your fat loss efforts by tapping into one of your body's natural mechanisms for unlocking and burning fat.

Ketosis is the metabolic state of the body when it has become adapted to burning fat instead of glucose as the primary fuel for energy.

Nutritional ketosis is induced by carbohydrate restriction while still eating moderate amounts of protein and liberal amounts of healthy fats and non-starchy vegetables. This practice allows you to receive all the necessary nutrition for optimal health.

Before I go into the details of how to transition into dietary ketosis, I want to talk about an example from the Bible from Jesus himself!

I firmly believe that Jesus began his three-year public ministry in the state of ketosis.

I know this because of this verse:

"And when He had fasted forty days and forty nights…"
(Matthew 4:2, NKJV).

In a fasted state, the body becomes adapted to burning fat for energy in just a few days. His mind was crystal clear and his body was clean and lean. He was spiritually and physically in a state of optimal health. He would be about His Father's business 24/7 for the next three years. He was a man on the go and constantly traveling on foot. He rarely slept in the same place.

I believe Jesus remained in ketosis until his death, and I believe this was a conscious decision on His part. He knew that he was at his optimal best in this state.

We know from reading the gospel that he ate fish, bread, and fruit. He drank water and some wine; and, of course, there was the Passover lamb. The fish was a great source of protein and healthy fat, full of omega 3, and free from mercury contamination.

I believe he would tell us today that we can enjoy optimal health if we leave highly processed bread, especially genetically modified organisms (GMOs) out of our diet!

Why?

The bread he ate in no way resembles the bread of our day. It was full of fiber and minimally processed from its natural state.

The fruit was much different from the hybrid, extra-large and super-sweet fruit of our day, which lacks the vitamins, minerals, and fiber content of the fruit of Jesus' day.

Jesus' enemies said of him that he was a "glutton and a winebibber, a friend of tax collectors and sinners" (Luke 7:34, NKJV).

"Jesus…a wino?" you may ask.

I don't think so, and neither do you, I'm sure.

I certainly cannot imagine Jesus eating like a pig turned loose in a modern-day buffet line. Was he a friend of sinners? Sure he was, but He was no glutton! Aren't you thankful that he was and still is a friend of sinners like you and me?

Let's talk about the wine Jesus occasionally drank. I grew up in the Bible Belt and I'm thankful I did. However, when I was a young Southern Baptist boy, I was taught that the wine Jesus drank at the wedding in Cana (see John 2:1-11) was grape juice.

Pretty absurd, I know!

Paul's advice to Timothy would have been a little absurd as well, if he told Timothy that a high fructose hit of grape juice was going to kill the bugs in his gut he had acquired from contaminated water (see 1 Timothy 5:23).

There is no doubt that the wine Jesus drank and Paul recommended, contained alcohol. However, I guarantee Jesus, Paul, and Timothy were not winos.

Personally, I believe a little wine for medicinal purposes or an occasional celebration is well within the moral conduct of a Christian.

However, drunkenness is always a sin and must be avoided (See Ephesians 5:18).

I believe Jesus stayed lean and strong throughout his very physically demanding ministry by remaining in ketosis. It gave him a steady flow of energy during his arduous days and long nights of prayer.

No one has ever lived who was more disciplined or in control of himself than Jesus. Paul said, "The fruit of the spirit is love, joy, peace...self control." (Gal. 5:22-23, NIV)

Temperance is, of course, self-control, and Jesus is the quintessential epitome of temperance. Can you imagine Jesus crashing every three hours and desperately needing a carb fix?

Food was a servant to Jesus. It served his nutritional needs, and that is exactly how we should view food as well.

That is not to say Jesus didn't enjoy eating. I'm sure he did. He was no servant to the demands of food, and his life was not dominated by thoughts of what he was going to eat.

I can't say I've always been the same. There was a time in my life when I lived to eat, instead of eating to live.

Food was always on my mind. What will I eat today and where will I eat today?

With only a few exceptions, food was my greatest source of pleasure. It was my reward for working and playing so hard.

I grew up in a middle-class family. My parents could not afford a new house, fancy car, or nice clothes, or any of the bells and whistles the rich folks had. However, we ate well and we ate often.

Our lives revolved around food. Maybe you can relate.

There was the traditional breakfast first thing in the morning, usually cereal during the week, and bacon and eggs with toast on the weekends. Breakfast was then followed by a mid-morning snack, usually a candy bar. That was followed by a lunch of hot dogs, chips, pop and cookies. The mid-afternoon snack was usually soda pop. Supper was the biggie. It was meat and tater time. Fried chicken, mashed potatoes and gravy, and canned sweet corn was followed by pie or cake with ice cream for dessert!

Just before bed, Dad and I had a big bowl of shredded wheat, with milk and several teaspoons of sugar.

All these meals were loaded with carbs and sugar in one form or another.

We ate lots of cereal made from grain, but we hardly ever had green vegetables or fruit.

We were just an average, American family eating a Standard American Diet high in starchy vegetables and grain products.

It had never occurred to me that the way farmers fatten up their cattle for market was to feed them lots of grain!

It was a pleasant surprise to learn that my weight problem, which resulted in my poor health, could be reversed. All I had to do was eliminate grain products, dairy, and beans, which were wreaking havoc with my digestion!

Pilgrims, I enjoy eating a good, home-cooked meal. My wife is the best cook in the world, and no, she didn't make me write that!

Note: Jesus' entry into ketosis was the result of doing a total fast of food. On average, this occurs in less than a week! However, anyone can enter into ketosis in three to four weeks by restricting carbohydrate consumption to 50 grams or less per day, and consuming adequate protein and healthy fats

On the Pilgrim's Plan, you will experience no hunger. You will have learned when to eat, what to eat and what not to eat to enjoy optimal health.

Now that I have introduced you to ketosis, the next chapter will answer the most common questions I get about this topic.

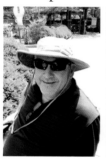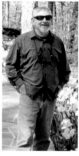

Brad: 40 pounds lost!
Seven months on my Keto journey and I'm down 40 pounds, off all diabetic medicine with an A1C of 5.1, blood pressure down taking half of one of my two blood pressure meds, triglycerides down to 145 from over 500.

I suffered from fatigue and brain fog that was so debilitating that some days to just get up out of my recliner was a challenge. Now I'm going to the YMCA three days a week doing aquacise and swimming.

Take control of your diet and you will take control of your health!
Brad

CHAPTER TEN

NUTRITIONAL KETOSIS: PART TWO

"Then he opened their minds so they could understand…"
(Luke 24:45, NIV).

Instead of a long chapter of me talking at you, I wanted to format this chapter in a way that addresses the most common questions about this phase.

This format will help you grasp the concepts quickly and prepare you for success as you move into converting your body to be a full-blown fat-burning machine.

Q: What is nutritional ketosis?

A: Ketosis is the metabolic state of the body when it has become adapted to burning fat instead of glucose as the primary fuel for energy. Nutritional ketosis is induced by carbohydrate restriction while still eating adequate amounts of protein, fat, and non-starchy vegetables. Thus, you receive all the nutrition necessary for optimal health.

Q: What does being a fat burner mean?

A: Being a fat burner means your body is now able to access your fat stores for use as your primary energy source. While in ketosis, our muscles are primarily fueled by free, fatty acids, and glycogen manufactured by our liver, but our brain and our hearts primarily are now running on the super-fuel known as ketones.

Q: What does being a sugar burner mean?
A: Being a sugar burner means your body is using carbohydrates/glucose as its primary fuel source for energy. In this metabolic state, you cannot access your fat reserves for fuel.

Q: How long can I stay in ketosis?
A: You can remain in a state of ketosis as long as you desire. Entire cultures have lived their entire lives in this metabolic state and enjoyed optimal health.

Q: What are ketones?
A: Ketones are the byproduct of fat metabolism, via the liver. They are derived from stored fat, which is a superior source of energy that our bodies use efficiently. Ketones are an anti-aging, slow, clean-burning source of energy. Ketones deliver a steady flow of energy all day long.

Q: How will my heart and brain respond to ketones?
A: Both heart and brain prefer ketones and perform more efficiently when using them. "The heart gets 28% more energy metabolizing beta-hydroxybutyrate (a ketone) than it does metabolizing glucose," Dr. Robert Veech.

There is no supplement or exercise routine capable of improving brain or heart function that outperforms ketones!

Q: Will ketosis limit my athletic performance?
A: The answer is no. Instead, it will enhance it. Remember, those who are in ketosis have far more endurance than sugar burners. Many professional athletes today are switching to ketone power versus glucose! Men like Kobe Bryant, Lebron James, and Sami Inkinen are just a few.

Professional bodybuilders who have always used ketosis in the cutting phase of their preparation for a show are now seeing it as a strategy to use year-round. They have learned to avoid the unhealthy bulking up stage they have traditionally employed.

Q: How long will it take for my body to enter ketosis and burn fat for energy?
A: On average, it takes 21 days of consuming 50 grams or less per day of carbohydrates to enter a state of ketosis. This is ample time for your body to up-regulate the enzymes necessary to properly metabolize and assimilate ingested fat, as well as convert stored fat into ketones.

Q: Will I experience any discomfort while going through the transition?
A: I personally had a symptom-free transition; however, some people report having a mild headache, constipation, lethargy, brain fog, dizziness, and leg cramping. When a person begins the way of eating detailed in this book, they will lose water before losing fat. The excess water leaving your body will take with it essential electrolytes, sodium, potassium, and magnesium, resulting in dehydration. This is the root cause of all the side effects of fat adaptation listed above. The cure is simple! Stay well hydrated and take a magnesium supplement. I personally use two products called 'Calm' and 'ZMA'. Any good health food store carries these products.

To insure your sodium levels are adequate, I recommend at least one teaspoon per day, and you may need to consume a cup of bullion or bone broth daily. I use Himalayan sea salt liberally to flavor my food. I also put just a pinch in my coffee. My potassium needs are primarily met by eating one avocado every day, plus supplementing with potassium citrate from Now Foods. Few people realize that an avocado has twice the potassium of a banana. If you do not like the taste of avocado, put it in a protein shake. It will make it thick and creamy, and you will not taste the avocado. By the way, if you experience strong urine odor or your breath smells like acetone (a sweet smell) during the transition phase, it will cease in a few weeks when you are fully adapted to burning fat as your primary energy source.

Q: Are there any pre-existing medical conditions that would make it unwise to pursue this strategy?
A: Type I diabetics should be very cautious and not attempt this unless they are under strict medical supervision. The danger is a condition called ketoacidosis. **Ketoacidosis can be fatal.**

However, many Type I diabetics are able to enter and remain in ketosis while under the supervision of their doctor. This is not an issue with Type II diabetics.

Ketosis is generally not recommended for pregnant women or children. They have unique nutritional needs that require higher carbohydrate consumption, which prevents them from entering into ketosis.

Q: How can I know if I am in ketosis?
A: A simple blood test you can do at home can tell you if you are in ketosis. A ketone meter can be found at any drug store. If it registers .5 mmol, you are in ketosis. Between 1 mmol and 5 mmol is the ideal reading. Most people in ketosis rarely go over 5 mmol. I personally have never been over 3 mmol.

If you don't have a ketone meter, the following are all indications that you are most likely in ketosis:

a. You can skip a meal or two and not experience any lack of energy.

b. You can work out in the gym on an empty stomach with no drop in your energy level.

c. You can sense your cognitive powers are returning as your memory is improving and your morning brain fog is a thing of the past.

d. Your sleep and mood greatly improves.

Q: What foods and supplements can speed up one's ability to reach ketosis?
A: MCT oil, coconut oil, and coconut milk will all help speed things up. MCT oil is especially good because it goes directly to the liver and quickly converts into ketone energy. Virtually all coconut products are ketogenic-friendly.

Q: Can a person live and thrive in a carbohydrate-restricted state of ketosis?
A: Carbohydrates are the one macronutrient that we can live without and still live well. This is not a theory, speculation, or some nutty hypothesis. Experts in the field of nutrition agree with this fact. According to the USDA, "The lower limit of dietary carbohydrate compatible with life apparently is zero, provided that adequate amounts of protein and fat are consumed."

However, I do not recommend a zero carb diet. For you to get all the nutrients you need for optimal health eating that kind of diet, you would need to consume what is called "offal", and awful stuff it is! Offal is the contents of the animal's stomach, essentially the pre-digested food that has not passed through the intestines, as well as the brains, heart, liver, kidneys, and testicles.

Therefore, I recommend you eat the most nutrient dense, non-starchy, mostly green vegetables you can while staying under 50 grams of carbs per day.

Q: Has any group of people ever lived in a state of ketosis as a way of life and maintained great health?
A: The Inuit Alaskan Eskimo and the Western Plains Indian enjoyed remarkably good health. The Eskimos live off of marine animals and land animals high in protein and fat. They had little to no access to carbohydrates, due to their very cold climate. The European explorers discovered the nomadic plains Indians were tall, handsome, and strong, as well as disease free. Their diet was primarily derived from the buffalo that roamed the plains by the millions. They also ate fish from the rivers and lakes and a few berries in the fall. Pemmican was their food in the dead of winter. It was made from buffalo fat and dried lean meat in a perfect ketosis blend of 80 percent fat and 20 percent protein. Both the Eskimo and Plains Indians fed their dogs the lean muscle meat and reserved the fattier cuts of meat for their own diet.

Q: What are the benefits of being in ketosis?
A: Here are some of the amazing benefits of nutritional ketosis:

• Your brain will function 28 percent more efficiently on ketones.

• You will experience less brain fog, and your memory will improve due to a 39% increase of blood flow to your brain. (PubMed)

• Your heart will perform up to 28 percent better on ketones, rather than glucose. Your energy will be steady throughout the day.

• You will not experience the carb-coma syndrome, or the up-and-down mood swings and irritability that accompany a carb crash.

• You will have greatly improved digestion, and no more heartburn, bloating, or excessive gas.

• You'll reach and maintain your ideal weight with ease.

• Your blood sugar and blood pressure will drop to normal levels.

• Your insulin levels will decrease, resulting in a longer, healthier life.

• Your triglyceride levels, the major indicator of cardiovascular disease, will go down significantly.

Q: Is it possible to gain weight while in ketosis?
A: If you are consuming more protein than is necessary for maintaining or building your muscle mass, the excess will be converted by your liver into fat and stored as such. Pilgrims, it is also possible, but **highly unlikely**, you could be in ketosis but consume more fat than you burn. If this happens, it will be stored in your adipose tissue!

Q: Can I gain muscle while in ketosis?
A: Yes, you can gain muscle through intense anaerobic exercise. Luis Villasenor has followed a ketogenic diet as a competition power-lifter and body builder for 16 years! A picture is worth a thousand words and his picture is the answer to the question. However, gaining muscle while

losing fat is very difficult! You will have to experiment with just how much extra protein and carbohydrates are enough to reach your goal, without kicking you out of ketosis.

Just look at the pictures blow of Luis and my sons Ken and Tony. They both lost over 30 pounds while in ketosis and were able to maintain and grow muscle during their transformations!

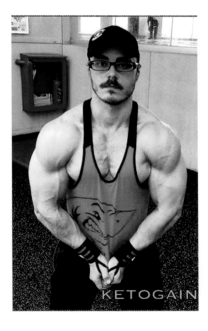
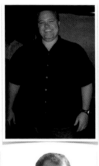
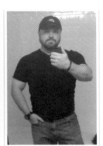
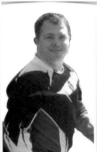
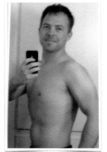

CHAPTER ELEVEN

FASTER RESULTS WITH INTERMITTENT FASTING

"When you fast…"
(Matthew 6:16, NKJV).

Intermittent fasting (or what some refer to as Time-Restricted Eating Plan) is another key tenet of my strategy. Once I became fat-adapted and was no longer primarily a sugar burner, I naturally could go 16-18 hours without being hungry. My body used my fat stores for energy. The benefits of fasting have been well established for thousands of years. The clearing effects it has on our minds and the cleansing effects on our bodies are indeed a marvel.

Jesus said, "**When** ye fast…," not **if** you fast. However, intermittent fasting is not the kind of fasting Jesus did. Jesus was sequestered during this time, and was praying in preparation for his public ministry. A 40-day fast for a working man or woman is not practical nor wise.

Intermittent fasting only requires you to fast a portion of each day.

Essentially, it amounts to skipping one meal per day. I am sure this is now sounding more doable to you and indeed, doable it is!

Several books have recently been written which document the extraordinary benefits of this type of fasting.

The least benefit is weight loss. **Eating all your meals within a six-to-eight hour window results in less inflammation.** This reduces diseases, which includes heart disease, cancer, stroke, and Alzheimer's.

You're probably thinking, "of course, if I only eat two meals per day I will naturally lose weight."

That does make sense, but with my plan and implementation of intermittent fasting, **a reduction in consumed calories is not necessary for fat loss. In fact, you may end up consuming more calories per day, not less!**

Here's why: fat has more than double the calories per gram than protein or carbohydrates! So, you may eat less volume of food on this plan, but your calorie intake may actually be higher. You will not be hungry, due to the satiating effect of high-quality fat and protein.

Intermittent fasting gives our bodies more time to rest and recuperate from the strain and stress of digestion and detoxification. Few people realize the energy required to digest food is one of our greatest, daily-energy drains.

You also may be thinking, "Pastor, I have always eaten breakfast and after all, Tony the Tiger says it is the most important meal of the day." There are many cereal/grain companies that sure hope you believe that and buy their products!

On the Pilgrim's Plan, **breakfast is the most important meal to skip!** Why? Because, we enter into fat-burning mode around six hours after our last meal the evening before. It is to your advantage to extend that fat-burning time a few more hours by waiting to eat your first meal around noon.

When intermittent fasting is combined with a ketogenic meal plan, it is not unreasonable to expect a three or four pound fat loss per week. This is especially true in the first few months!

Replace Your Breakfast With This…
If you find that you need an energy boost in the morning to start your day, I have the answer, and it is downright miraculous.

It is called Bulletproof Coffee and is the brainchild of a guy named Dave Asprey. It is made with coffee, real butter, and a special kind of natural oil called Medium Chain Triglyceride (MCT), which is a purified form of coconut oil.

Note: you may be wondering why I am talking about a breakfast here when we are supposed to be fasting 16-18 hours a day! The reason is that fat via MCT oil or butter, when consumed without protein or carbohydrates, does not raise your blood sugar levels. Therefore, there is no insulin release from your pancreas to trigger storage of fat in your fat cells. Thus, it is burned for energy or eliminated. This is why you can consume this particular drink for breakfast without stopping ketone production, thereby staying in ketosis.

I like to think of it as pure energy. Unlike other fat sources that require a lengthy process of metabolism, **MCT oil goes directly to your liver, via the portal vein. The liver promptly converts it to ketone energy.**

MCT oil yields energy as fast as simple carbohydrates, but without an insulin spike. There is no high/low roller coaster ride. You will experience a steady flow of energy. Excess ketones, unlike carbohydrates/glucose, are not stored. They are eliminated through your lungs, through your urine, and through your stool!

How much MCT oil should you consume? I recommend starting with a teaspoon first thing in the morning. I like putting it in a cup of coffee with a teaspoon of real butter for an extra turbocharged experience! However, if you are not a coffee drinker, tea works just as well. It is the synergistic effect of the MCT oil, real butter, and caffeine from the coffee that produces the smooth and sustained energy release throughout the day.

I just add the MCT Oil and real butter to my morning coffee and stir it up with a spoon, but if you will take the time to put them in blender you will experience the most delicious latte you ever drank! If you like, you may even sweeten it a bit with Stevia.

When break time rolls around at work, have another cup of turbocharged coffee, and you will be good to go until lunch. Over the next few weeks you could gradually increase from one teaspoon at a time to two teaspoons. Eventually, you could use one tablespoon each time. This goes for the butter too.

Why ease into this? For some people a tablespoon at a time will result in loose bowels or full-blown diarrhea. I began with a tablespoon of MCT oil and butter, and never experienced any negative symptoms. Some of my friends were not so blessed!

Because Bulletproof Coffee has such a satiating effect upon your appetite, I do not recommend you consume more than two of them per day!

You only eat two meals and a snack, **if you need it**, on the Pilgrim's Plan.

Remember, even though you are compressing these two meals and a snack into a six to eight hour window, you are not compromising on the amount of calories or the quality of food that you are eating. You will think you are eating like a king or queen once you get started and begin to experience the power of delicious, real food.

What about a full food fast?
If you desire to do a total food fast for two to three days for spiritual or physical reasons, it will do you good on every level. It will clear your mind, cleanse your body, and strengthen your spirit when combined with prayer. Some folks take a few days of vacation time every year and fast. This type of fast is a proven way to lower your homeostatic set point, which results in you being healthy at a lower weight. Fasting is also an excellent way to break through a plateau in your weight loss.

Once you have mastered intermittent fasting and experience its benefits, I predict you will never again go back to the cereal/grain company's recommendation.

Bacon and eggs are just as good at noon, which is why you can get them at most restaurants any time of day.

Praise the Lord!

SECTION FIVE:

LIFESTYLE CHANGES

FOR OPTIMAL HEALTH

CHAPTER TWELVE

SLEEP:
YOUR SECRET WEAPON
AGAINST FAT

"Jesus was in the stern, sleeping on a cushion"
(Mark 4:38, NIV).

Everyone has burned the candle at both ends, and discovered how it was really counter-productive. We must have adequate sleep in order to be at our best. Sleep defragments our organic computer (our brain) of all the clutter that has entered it through the day. We wake up and our minds are fresh, sharp, and clear. We are ready for thousands of new bits of information that will come our way that day.

During the night, our major organs get a much-needed rest as our hearts beat slower, and the digestive system takes a break. Our muscles relax from the labors of the day. In a sense, we are reborn every morning. Like the birds outside our windows, we begin to chirp and sing, "This is the day, this is the day that the Lord has made…" (Psalm 118:24, KJV).

I am sure there are many good reasons why our Lord made the night as well as the day. Perhaps none is greater than to get us to slow down, rest, sleep, and rejuvenate our mind and body.

Sleep isn't just important; it's paramount to achieving optimal health.

Generally speaking, eight hours of sleep is adequate. You may get by on a little less or require a little more, depending on your age, health, and activity level.

The important thing to note, is that the quality of your sleep is more important than the number of hours you get.

No doubt you have spent a sleepless night, tossing and turning and have awakened just as tired, as when you went to bed. Many factors, including worry, stress, pain, sickness, and noise, played a role in your sleepless night.

Here are some suggestions for a good night's rest:

Don't consume any caffeinated drink after midday.
It is hard to sleep when you are bouncing off the walls. Your central nervous system needs enough time to wind down to allow for a good night's rest.

Plan your last meal of the day at least three hours before bed.
You will sleep better on an empty stomach rather than one that is working hard to digest a heavy meal.

Turn off the TV and shut down the computer after your evening meal.
Your nervous system needs to have reduced stimuli for up to two hours prior to falling asleep. This ensures that your mind is calm and ready to fall into deep, restorative sleep.

Take a 15-minute evening walk.
The fresh air will do you good. This will also help settle your evening meal and aid digestion.

Spend some quality time with your family.
Sharing the day's activities and tomorrow's plans is a wise way to end your day. Be sure to pray for and bless them at the conclusion of these meaningful conversations.

Take a hot shower or sit in the tub
Some Epsom salts added to the water will help relax and detox your body. Epsom salts contains magnesium, which is very effective for relaxing the muscles and helps bring relief from arthritis and joint pain. People flock to spas for the relaxing benefits of the sulfur and magnesium-rich waters of hot springs. You might also have some soft praise and worship music in the background. Don't fall asleep in the tub or else you will awaken looking like a wrinkled prune!

Turn your thermostat below 70 degrees.
You will sleep much better in a cool room. Something happens to us when the room we sleep in is a bit cool, but not cold. Our bodies seem to do better and stay in deep sleep longer, due to the cooler temperatures.

Keep your bedroom as dark as possible.
Light from computers, TVs, clocks, and night-lights have been proven to negatively affect the quality of your sleep. I even recommend dark, thick curtains that block all light in order to create total darkness in your room.

Pray yourself to sleep
When you are ready to sleep, begin counting your blessings in prayer. Be sure to express your gratitude for God's amazing grace in restoring your health.

CHAPTER THIRTEEN

HOW STRESS MAKES YOU FAT

"The worries of life…"
(Mark 4:19, NIV).

You may be wondering what stress has to do with regaining your health and reaching your ideal weight. Stress releases cortisol which shuts down fat burning immediately.

In Mark 4:19, Jesus explains that worry is counterproductive. The more you worry about the cares of this world, the more you will be hindered in your ability to be fruitful in your pursuit of your goal of honoring God and His word by fulfilling your mission upon earth!

How well you transition to the Pilgrim's Plan way of eating will depend in large part upon how well you handle stress, and the adversity you will face.

Your first month will be your make or break month. Charlie Rich was right when he sang, "Life has its little ups and downs, like ponies on a merry-go-round." This is just a natural part of life that we understand as Christians.

When you become stressed, whether in spirit, soul, or body, your brain automatically signals the body to release cortisol. Cortisol is known as the fight-or-flight hormone, which helps protect you and me "from lions and tigers and bears, oh my!"

Cortisol signals the liver to break down glycogen, which is stored in the liver and turn it into glucose. Your liver then releases that glucose into the bloodstream for a rush of energy to run fast or fight for your life. It is amazing how God created our bodies to survive any adverse condition we might face!

However, as you now understand, having spikes of glucose in your bloodstream is not conducive to fat loss! As long as we are burning glucose for energy, we are not burning fat for energy.

When we are in stress mode, we cannot burn fat from our fat depots! **Being under a lot of stress makes it close to impossible to lose fat.**

What happens if there is no immediate danger to our lives?

There is no wild animal chasing us, or a possible ambush from a soldier in a combat zone.

What if we are stressed in our soul, and our brain has sent the signal to start the hormonal response?

When the high blood sugar rush is over, we experience low blood sugar. We are hungry and head for the refrigerator!

This is how stress defeats us in our goal to lose fat!

However, don't make the mistake of thinking cortisol or any other God-given hormone is your enemy. Our hormones are operating just as God designed them. Stress is the enemy that must be defeated, or it will defeat you at every level—spirit, soul, and body!

Pilgrim, we are living with situations all around us that have the potential to raise our stress levels.

Our Bible never hid this fact from us. Jesus said, "In this world ye shall have tribulation: but be of good cheer, I have overcome the world" (John 16:33, NKJV). And Pilgrim, you will overcome, "Because greater is He that is in you than he who is in the world" (1 John 4:4, NKJV).

Tribulation, troubles, trials, and sorrows certainly create stress in our lives. Job said, "Yet man is born to trouble, as the sparks fly upward" (Job 5:7, NKJV). No one has ever been exempt from the pressures of life! We have no choice but to deal with it. From the cradle to the coffin, it is ours to face.

The question is, how are you going to deal with it?

The answer is not found in a bottle of booze, a pill, needle, or your refrigerator! You cannot ignore it. It will not go away. You will either master it, or it will master you.

The Ultimate Stress Buster: Prayer
"Now in the morning, having risen a long while before daylight, He went out and departed to a solitary place; and there he prayed" (Mark 1:35, NKJV).

"Jesus often withdrew to lonely places and prayed." (Luke 5:16, NIV)

"He… continued all night in prayer to God" (Luke 6:12, NIV).

Pilgrims, no one has ever been more stressed than Jesus on the night of His betrayal. How did He handle the enormous pressure of that dreadful night? He prayed and God answered His prayer!

"And there appeared an angel unto Him from heaven, strengthening Him" (Luke 22:43, KJV).

From that moment forward, Jesus was fully prepared to finish His mission on earth! His last words on the cross were, "It is finished" (John 19:30, KJV). Pilgrims, please understand that **prayer is the key to overcoming stress.**

Through prayer, you will be able to achieve your goal, just as Jesus achieved his. Do not underestimate the power of prayer to see you through this journey.

Communing with God one-on-one was vitally important to Jesus. Prayer calms our anxieties and fears and brings peace to our troubled souls. It is in prayer that we find inspiration, fresh anointing, and guidance through life's maze.

In 1845, William W. Walford wrote the following beautiful hymn that talks about the importance of prayer:

"Sweet Hour of Prayer."
Sweet hour of prayer! Sweet hour of prayer!
That calls me from a world of care
And bids me at my Father's throne
Make all my wants and wishes known.
In seasons of distress and grief
My soul has often found relief,
And oft escaped the tempter's snare,
By thy return, sweet hour of prayer!

Paul said, "Don't worry about anything, instead, pray about everything. Tell God what you need, and thank Him for all He has done. Then you will experience God's peace, which exceeds anything we can understand. His peace will guard your hearts and minds as you live in Christ Jesus" (Phil. 4:6-7, NLT).

Paul practiced what he preached. When he was under stress, the Bible records that, "But at midnight Paul and Silas were praying and singing hymns unto God..." (Acts 16:25, NKJV) In pain and in prison, Paul had peace through the greatest panacea a Christian can have, prayer and praise.

Pilgrims, pray your way through this journey to restored health. Don't worry because there is a new you coming very soon.

Your prayers will be answered and your miraculous transformation will be the proof.

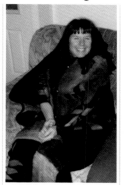 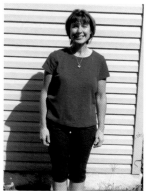

Marianne Morris: 39 Pounds Lost!

This book was so helpful to me. I have gone from 204 pounds to 165. The wonderful thing is it came off my middle.

I was a tight 14 women's, and now I wear a size 10, and am able to wear an 8 in some things.

I would recommend this book for anyone who wants to lose the weight and feel good.

God Bless you Pastor Dennis!!!!

I am praying for the success of this book.

Marianne Morris

CHAPTER FOURTEEN

EXERCISE...NOT REQUIRED BUT BENEFICIAL!

"As the saying goes...exercise is good for your body"
(1 Timothy 4:8, CEV).

There are only two ways you can remain a "sugar burner" and lose weight. Neither way is healthy. One is a calorie-restricted diet, which leaves you lethargic, hungry, and grumpy. The other is an obsessive and strenuous exercise regimen, which puts you at risk for injury and stresses your body. It can cause a massive release of cortisol and can throw your fat burning hormones out of balance, thus stopping your fat loss dead in its tracks.

Either one, or a combination of the two, will work short term. Neither is sustainable long term, and failure is inevitable.

It's the old two-step song and dance of "eat less and exercise more" that we have heard repeatedly from the medical community. If that tired tune worked, would we have an obesity epidemic?

Why 'Eat Less' Doesn't Work
Starvation diets slow down our metabolism and the rate of fat-burning, because our bodies think we are starving and preserves what energy we have left.

Starvation diets also leave us hungry and miserable. We inevitably fall off the wagon and head to the nearest buffet line (my wife likes to call them "troughs").

Why 'Exercise More' Doesn't Work

"Exercise stimulates an increase in appetite and calorie consumption such that it results in a wash when it comes to weight management." Mark Sisson

Exercise is actually a very inefficient way to lose weight!

Fortunately, there is a way to lose fat without exercise, and you never have to be hungry.

The secret is to change your primary energy source from sugar/glucose to fat/ketones.

The Proper Use Of Exercise Is Maintenance

Exercise relates to this plan, but it depends upon several factors like your age, overall health and ability to exercise.

When I began this journey, I was 80 pounds overweight and had very little energy. My blood pressure was extremely high and I was tired all the time. For me, exercise was not an option. In fact, **I lost all my excess fat without exercise on this plan.**

As I mentioned earlier in this book, the first thing I did when I started my weight loss journey was to cancel my YMCA membership! I knew that working out and stressing my body at the gym would cause me to be very tired, stressed, and also spike my hunger levels. Clearly this was not what I wanted.

However, if you are able to exercise, it will speed up your progress, if it is done correctly.

Here is a simple illustration. If you start your car and let it run, it will burn gasoline at a minimal rate. But if you get into the car and slowly drive around the block, it will burn gas at a higher rate. Merge onto the freeway and put the pedal to the metal. You can see the fuel gauge decreasing at an accelerating rate, no pun intended. I'm sure you get the point.

If exercise is something you haven't done in a while, don't sweat it! Well, actually, a little sweat would help, but no need to run a marathon.

The best exercise of all time is walking!

Walking outside in the fresh air is best, and early morning or late evening is prime time. I suggest 20 minutes, three days per week. If the weather is bad, I have a Schwinn Airdyne bike in my office that I use.

Hit It Pilgrims!
With High Intensity Interval Training (HIIT)

Once you have advanced beyond the stage of just walking or riding the bike at a slow, easy pace and are healthy and physically able, I highly recommend high intensity interval training. This style of exercise is great because it burns up to nine times more fat than traditional aerobic training. This has been scientifically proven by Laval University in Canada, as well as Colorado State University and other reputable organizations.

HIIT yields the best benefits of aerobic and anaerobic workouts in an economy of time! Here's how it works. With HIIT, you go all out with an intense exercise like sprinting or burpees for a short period of time (30 seconds), which is followed by a brief rest period (1 minute). This cycle is repeated 7 times (depending on your fitness level), and you are done! I recommend you do this three times per week.

I use my dual-action Schwinn Airdyne Bike for this type of training exercise. It gives me a great upper and lower body workout in 10.5 minutes with the least possibility of injury!

Before you begin HIIT, you should do ten minutes of stretching exercises to warm up.

When you're physically able and want to gain muscle mass, you can start lifting weights. Remember that proper form is critical in order to prevent injury. Therefore, I highly recommend you seek the assistance of a certified trainer. Twenty minutes, three times per week is enough. Start light, and then gradually increase the resistance each week. On your last repetition, lower the weight as slowly as you can for optimal results.

Allow yourself 48 hours between weight-training sessions, which allows your body to heal and repair itself. **You can train at home.** However, the YMCA, a good friendly Christian-based facility, will have excellent trainers to assist you in proper form while lifting weights. They also have excellent group-sporting activities available such as basketball, volleyball, soccer, racquetball, and pickleball. Swimming and other water aerobics are also excellent forms of exercise.

It has been said that the best exercise is the one you enjoy doing and will do often. For me, it is basketball!

I play three or four times per week, in addition to my regular aerobic and anaerobic routine. Remember this wise quote from Oliver Wendell Holmes, **"Men do not quit playing because they grow old; they grow old because they quit playing!"**

Exercise is an excellent way to help you maintain your weight loss.

The health benefits of cardio and weight training are many, but you **cannot exercise your way out of a bad diet.**

It breaks my heart to see so many people on a treadmill going nowhere, just sweating away. They will never arrive at their destination.

I was once one of them!

Then I learned the secret to unlocking my fat stores, which had nothing to do with exercise!

Pilgrims, transforming your body is 80 percent diet. Remember, six pack abs are made in the kitchen, not the gym!

Remember, **you don't have to exercise at all on this plan in order to lose fat!**

If you can exercise do it intelligently but don't expect exercise to be the mechanism behind your weight loss. It simply isn't and that is a scientific fact.

Pilgrims, two hours per week is not excessive is it? Aim for 20 minutes per day, Monday through Saturday.

Sunday is the Lord's Day, so spend it with Him and your family.

CHAPTER FIFTEEN

THE TRUTH ABOUT SUPPLEMENTS

"Make every effort to supplement your faith"
(2 Peter 1:5, ESV).

Fellow Pilgrims! Pills, powders, and potions are far from being the best way to get all the vitamins, minerals, and antioxidants your body requires for optimal health. If you eat according to the guidelines laid out in this book, you won't have much need for supplements.

Most, but **not all,** multivitamins and performance-enhancing supplements are a complete waste of your hard-earned money.

A good health food store has natural herbal remedies and organic, locally raised honey. They may offer produce, meat, and dairy products from grass-fed cows, plus free-range chickens and their eggs. These stores are a tremendous asset to any community.

However, I do recommend a few supplements that you may begin taking immediately. I do not believe that today's food supply provides adequate supplies of certain particular vitamins, minerals, and oils.

The supplements that make my must have list are:

Omega-3, Vitamin D3, ZMA, Magnesium, Turmeric/Curcumin, Digestive Enzymes, and MCT Oil.

Let's look at each one in more detail.

Omega-3

If you are eating salmon or sardines high in omega-3, two to three times per week, you can forgo this supplement. Salmon or sardines are excellent sources of this essential, fatty acid. Just make sure the salmon is not farm raised, because wild-caught fresh or canned Alaskan salmon is the best choice.

One way or another, you must get this essential fatty acid into your body. Your heart and brain will thank you. Omega-3s can reduce sudden cardiac death by 50-80 percent! One to two grams per day is all that is necessary.

Personally, my memory recall was turbocharged when I began using the combination of an Omega-3 product AND feeding my brain ketones via the ketogenic diet described in this book.

Some people don't like taking fish oil capsules since many Omega-3 fish oil capsules on the market are of inferior quality and can create a fishy tasting burp! If you cannot find a high quality fish oil capsule, then I recommend a product called Vectomega. I guarantee you will not have "fish burps" with this product.

If you choose to get your Omega-3 oils strictly from your diet, and also chose to not eat fish for fear of mercury contamination, organic free range chicken eggs and grass-fed beef provide alternate choices.

D3

More than 90 percent of Americans are vitamin D3-deficient.

Vitamin D3 is called the "sunshine vitamin", since our bodies generate it from sunlight absorbed into the skin. You may ask yourself "Why do I need this supplement?" Practically speaking, we live in houses, drive our cars to work, and sit behind a desk all day. Then we drive home, go inside, and repeat the process day after day. The main function of this vitamin is to regulate the absorption of calcium in our bones to prevent rickets. This supplement is especially needed in the winter months, but some people will need it all year long. Pilgrims, it is a very inexpensive supplement, and its benefits may save your life. Personally, I take 5,000 I.U. per day from Now Foods.

Other benefits of vitamin D3 include, but are not limited to..:

- •Greatly reduce inflammation.
- • Helps prevent most forms of cancer.
- • Helps prevent autoimmune diseases.
- • Supports a healthy immune system.
- • Helps prevent cardiovascular disease.
- • Helps prevent Parkinson's disease.
- • Helps support brain health.

ZMA

I also recommend a combination supplement called ZMA. ZMA is a supplement that contains Zinc, Magnesium and vitamin B6.

Zinc is a powerful antioxidant and immune booster. Zinc also detoxifies the brain of heavy metals, thus guarding against Alzheimer's disease.

Of interest to men, Zinc is also shown to increase testosterone in males, who are deficient in this hormone.

Note: vitamin B6 and Magnesium also aid zinc in the absorption and conversion of free cholesterol to testosterone.

Magnesium is a great muscle relaxer, thus aiding sleep. It is estimated 80 percent of Americans are deficient in this essential mineral. Your heart health is dependent upon adequate magnesium supplementation! This mineral is required for over 300 critical biological processes in the human body!

On a ketogenic diet, one must keep this electrolyte (magnesium) in an optimal range. An electrolyte imbalance is the major cause of brain fog, headaches, dizziness, constipation, lethargy, and muscle cramps. I use 'Now Sports' product just before I go to bed.

Magnesium
When a person begins the way of eating as detailed in this book, you will lose water before you begin to lose fat. The excess water leaving your body will take with it essential electrolytes, sodium, potassium, and magnesium. The result is dehydration. This is the root cause of all the side effects of fat adaptation listed above. The cure is simple! Stay well hydrated and take a magnesium supplement. My wife uses a product called 'Calm' just before bed.

Turmeric / Curcumin
Turmeric helps control blood sugar and removes plaque from your brain that can lead to Alzheimer's. It also reduces inflammation associated with arthritis and helps prevent

cancer! Be sure to use a product that contains black pepper extract to guarantee absorption. I use the brand 'Stop Aging Now' curcumin 2k formula 1330 mg with BioPerine.

Digestive Enzymes

This supplement is very helpful to insure proper digestion, especially if you have had your gallbladder removed or if you are a senior citizen. Be sure to buy one that has ox bile in it! I use a product from Now Foods called Super Enzymes. It is inexpensive, and I highly recommend it to ensure proper digestion, especially while adapting to a high-fat diet.

MCT Oil

Technically this is not a supplement, but I want to mention MCT Oil here because of its importance to your success on this program. This is especially true in the first few months of becoming fat adapted. Once you are fully adapted to burning fat for your primary energy source, you would not actually need this supplement, unless you want to keep enjoying the smooth energy delivery and appetite suppression that it provides.

In addition, if you love your Bulletproof Coffee, there is nothing wrong with continuing your use of it. I still love Bulletproof Coffee and always will! This really helped me in my transition from a sugar burner to a fat burner. Thank you very much, Dave Asprey!

I use Now Foods 32 ounce MCT oil.

SECTION SIX:

THE MASTER KEY

CHAPTER SIXTEEN

HOW TO GUARANTEE YOUR SUCCESS

"…write the vision and make it plain on tablets"
(Habakkuk 2:2, NKJV).

Now that you understand how you have been misled when it comes to nutrition, it is time to turn your attention inward and decide exactly what you want to accomplish with your health.

This chapter is one of the most valuable in the entire book for those who are wise and ready to apply its nuggets of wisdom.

Take time to read and follow this chapter's progression, and I guarantee it will greatly improve your results.

If you will study this chapter and apply its wisdom, then your success is almost guaranteed!

Pilgrims, when you want to accomplish something important, there are five major factors that will be crucial to your success.

These five factors are…

Purpose:
What is your Vision? What do you want and why do you want it?

Passion:
How bad do you want it? Do you want it as much as your next breath?

Plan:
Do you have a plan? Yes! This book is the plan!

Pursue:
Are you willing to take action and do whatever it takes as you pursue your goal?

Prayer:
A faith filled prayer confirming God's promises produces positive results and the good book says, "Delight thyself also in the Lord; and he shall give thee the desires of thine heart" (Psalm 37:4, KJV).

Now let's dig into each one of these five factors a little deeper.

Purpose
The very first thing I want you to do is to take out a clean sheet of paper and grab a pen or pencil. You will begin your Pilgrim's Plan journey by writing your specific goals on this journey.

Did you know that those who write their goals and review them daily are 80 percent more likely to succeed? Study after study has confirmed this! The very act of writing your specific fat loss goal down in detail will dramatically increase the likelihood that you achieve your goal.

Go ahead and write your goals down now. Simply write out in plain English what you want to accomplish with your health.

Next, use the **Three Step Bulletproof Goal Setting** process to ensure that you stay on track.

Step One: Know Your 'Reason Why'
Knowing the deep emotional reason why you want to lose weight can provide an endless source of motivation to you.

Why are you REALLY embarking upon this journey?

Is it just to lose some extra fat off your body, or does it go deeper than that?

Do you want to regain your health so that you can be a better husband/wife, parent, brother, sister, or servant of the Lord?

Is your extra weight keeping you from doing things that you want to do?

Take time to dig into this question Pilgrims, I want you to keep asking the question, "Why must I lose this fat?" Keep asking until you get to the deep, underlying emotional reason why.

This reason why is the real reason you are reading this book today.

You may not truly know what it is at this very moment, but if you sit down in a quiet spot and keep asking that question until the tears start to roll, you will discover it. I promise.

Step Two: Create a vivid picture
Once you know your reason why, be very specific in how

you write down your Vision of your new self. Be courageous and bold and state exactly what you want. It must represent exactly what you are aiming for. Take dead aim, Pilgrim!

I cannot over-emphasize the fact you must have a specific target you're aiming for or you will soon lose your motivation and abandon your journey!

Imagine a picture of you at your optimal level of health and fitness.

Now, describe exactly how you will look in your new body.

Next, describe how you would feel after you have finally lost all the fat that has been holding you back over the years.

THIS is what you can achieve and will achieve if you truly want it.

Step Three: Ask yourself the right question everyday! Our minds are one of the most powerful gifts the good Lord gave us. We can use our minds to help us stay on track, solve problems, and stay motivated. The key is to ask the right questions. This especially applies to weight loss, and it's quite simple to do.

Just write the question below on to a note card and tape it to your bathroom mirror. Every morning I want you to ask yourself one simple question.

The Question:

"As I'm effortlessly implementing the Pilgrim's Plan, how can I find even more enjoyable ways to prepare and eat healthy food?"

That's it!

Everything begins in the mind before it ever materializes in the physical realm.

It's true that "What you think about comes about!"

Even the Bible agrees, "For as he thinketh in his heart so is he", says the preacher (Proverbs 23:7, KJV).

If you will commit to asking yourself the question shown above every morning (and more often if you can) for the next 30 days, you will be surprised how easy it will be to think of better food choices. In fact, you will start to notice better options no matter where you are.

Next, I want you to tape your goals somewhere you will see it every day.

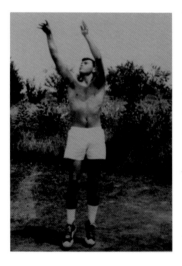

Next to your goals, tape a picture of yourself when you were at your best. Mine was a picture of myself shooting a basketball, with my arms high in the air. I was 19 years old when the picture was taken I was enjoying optimal health and abundant energy! That image was exactly my goal when I embarked upon this journey!

At this point you should have the following items in place:

1. Your own Vision in detail of what you want to look like.

2. Your daily question written out on a note card.

3. A picture of you (or someone you admire) that represents a visual image of what you want to look like.

I wanted to feel like that lively young man again shooting baskets. I visualized it, dreamed about it, and in less than one year, I became that person once again. I did so by following "The Pilgrim's Plan" outlined in this book and by utilizing the motivation strategies shared in this chapter.

This simple Three Step Bulletproof Goal Setting process that I just taught you is going to be a huge advantage to you! It is powerful, so use it wisely!

Passion
Now, in addition to intent, **there is a second element** critical to your success.

That element is **passion**.

"PASSION CREATES THE DESIRE AND THE COURAGE TO DO WHATEVER IT TAKES TO ACHIEVE YOUR GOAL." The Pilgrim

You must possess a burning passion with a fire burning inside you that will not be quenched until you are that person in the mirror. From that passion, you will find the energy to overcome every obstacle that stands in your way.
Whether you win or lose this challenge, it all comes down to how badly you really want it. Are you passionate about it? Are you excited about the possibilities of your goal? Is your heart in it 100 percent? If so, you will reach your goal!

After all, it is just a matter of time, and time passes so quickly, doesn't it? Soon, you are going to need a new wardrobe. You'll need new pictures, so you can forever put away the old ones, where you looked so tired and unhealthy. Or, you could keep those pictures around to remind yourself that the conventional wisdom of our so-called health experts almost destroyed your health.

Pilgrims, everyone has a destiny to fulfill.

A mission, if you will.

A calling in life.

A sense of responsibility.

A job to do!

Jesus said in Luke 19:13 that we were "to occupy until I come." In other words, stay busy, be productive, be active, be profitable! Paul said in 2 Timothy 4:7, NKJV, "I have fought the good fight, I have finished the race, I have kept the faith."

How about you my friend? Have you finished the race or **have you been sidelined with diet-related health issues?**

Pilgrims, it is not too late to get well and get back into fulfilling your destiny.

I believe your best days are ahead of you!

Rise up men and women of God and reclaim your health to the glory of the God who created you in His image!

Pilgrims, you must have an open and willing mind!

Six years ago, I knew my life's work was not done. I began with an open mind and a willing mind to do whatever it would take to regain my health. I was willing to read and heed the book my son gave me!

God had given me the knowledge I needed to regain my health and the wisdom to apply that knowledge. I was now physically able to pursue my mission in life, unhindered by poor health!

Oh Pilgrims, I pray you will follow my example and come along beside me on this journey and experience the same life extension that I have. I now have a life full of abundant energy and unspeakable joy.

You have a **purpose, passion,** and now, with this book, you have a **plan.**

Plan
The third factor is your Plan. As we mentioned earlier, this book IS your plan. The Pilgrim's Plan is the exact system I used to lose over 80 pounds, and you can too! Be sure to read this book two or three times to make sure you pick up all the nuggets of wisdom.

Pursue
Now comes the most critical factor. This is where the rubber meets the road. You must pursue your goal and be willing to do what others won't, in order to achieve what others don't!

Remember this saying:
"The difference between who you are and who you want to be is what you do!"
Bill Phillips

Be willing to do whatever it will take to achieve optimal health, energy, and freedom from prescription drugs.

Here is where "Woulda-coulda-shoulda" must become, "I did it."

You must **pursue** your objective like someone with his or her hair on fire, sprinting for a pond!

The truth is, the Pilgrim's Plan will only work if you work at it!

"Faith without works is dead!" (James 2:26 KJV)

"But be doers of the word, and not hearers only, deceiving yourselves" (James 1:22, NKJV).

As you go through the Pilgrim's Plan, craft a list of what your path will require of you. As I mentioned earlier, my miracle began when I was willing to commit to the plan laid out in this book! I was never hungry and ate plenty of delicious food every day.

However, I did have to commit to changing my old patterns. **Pilgrims, for things to change, some things have to change!** There is no way around that fact!

If, after reviewing the list, you may say to yourself, "I could not do this or give up that." If that is the case, then you must resign yourself to living as you are now!
The sad truth is things will get much worse than they are now unless you are willing to **take full responsibility for your health.** You must make this uncompromising commitment to **do whatever it takes.**

Prayer

God calls those things that do not exist as though they did. (see Romans 4:17 NKJV) As a child of God, you should do likewise.

"You will pronounce something to be, and He will make it so; light will break out across all your paths" (Job 22:28, The Voice).

In prayer to your heavenly father and in the name of Jesus, declare with unwavering faith that you will achieve your goal by His grace, and favor upon your life, knowing it is His will that you be in good health! (see 3 John 1:2, NKJV)

Summary

Now that you understand the five key factors that will guarantee your success on this journey, let's turn our attention to another very important concept.
That concept is your level of desire.

How bad do you want to change your health?

CHAPTER SEVENTEEN

YOU GOTTA WANT IT!

"When you seek me, you will find me,
provided you seek for me wholeheartedly"
(Jeremiah 29:13, CJB).

Let us consider that important verse I quoted earlier, Proverbs 23:7, "For as he thinketh in his heart, so is he."

The general interpretation of that verse is what you think about will come about.

Pilgrim, if you are a believer like me, you believe every word of the Bible is true. But, I know that not everything I have thought about has come about. I'm not sure about you, but I'm thankful for this!

So, is the verse true or not?

I believe it is true when we understand the essence of what it means. It is not saying that everything you think about will come about. The key to understanding this verse is in the three words, "in his heart."

What is meant by that phrase is what you think about **passionately,** in your heart, will come about.

It also means that which we think about continually, comes about.

When we think about something passionately and meditate on it daily, we move even closer to its manifestation.

What's in your heart is very important to you. When it burns passionately within you, you become emotionally connected to it. As you meditate upon your goal, you just naturally gravitate toward it and it toward you! Believe me when I say it's on its way to becoming a reality in your life. It's just a matter of time.

Psalm 37:4, (KJV) says, "Delight thyself also in the Lord and He shall give thee the desires of thine heart."

By simply opening this book, you expressed a desire to regain your health and be able to live without prescription medicine and its awful side effects.

Jesus said that nothing is impossible with God, and we all know that is true. But did you know He also said, "nothing shall be impossible unto you?" (See Luke 1:37, Matthew 17:20 and Mark 9:23)

Did Jesus truly mean it's possible for you to be restored to optimal health? You know the answer to that question.

Friend, it is God's will that you, "Prosper and be in health, even as thy soul prospereth" (3 John 2, KJV). The great apostle Paul prayed for his fellow Thessalonian Christians "…and I pray God your whole spirit and soul and body be preserved blameless unto the coming of our Lord Jesus Christ." (1 Thessalonians 5:23, KJV)

CHAPTER EIGHTEEN

METAMORPHOSIS

"Be not conformed to this world but be ye transformed by the
renewing of your mind, that you may prove what is that good,
and acceptable and perfect, will of God"
(Romans 12:2, KJV).

We have talked about the heart and its passionate goal
that burns within us. Now, let's talk about the mind.

The context of the verse at the top of this chapter is
about becoming a new person in Christ by changing the
way we think, otherwise, we cannot experience God's
perfect will for our lives.

This is accomplished by reading, believing, and applying
the counsel in God's word.

If we do so, we will go through a transformation. The
word in Greek is **metamorphosis.** It will literally change
you into a different person.

We see this when a caterpillar, through the miracle of
metamorphosis, becomes a butterfly. Another example from nature is when the lowly tadpole becomes the
proud bullfrog.

We become like our Lord as we read and heed the Word.
It is a gradual process (See 2 Corinthians 3:18).

Pilgrim, you desire to become a new person, so let us
apply this verse to that goal as well.

The takeaway from this verse is the first phrase, **"Be not conformed to this world."**

Conformity to the health guidelines of this world has not gone well for you or anyone else. The transformation you are about to undergo takes place first in your mind.

Perhaps you have realized, out of necessity, **that it is time to change the way you think about food.**

Pilgrim, you are what you eat! What you should eat, why, and when you should eat it are all questions I have answered in this book.

Some changes in your health will occur during the first week. Other changes will occur after a few weeks and still others in a few months. You will be amazed a year from now at your transformation.

Remember, **patience** is a Christian virtue (see Galatians 5:22-23).

Paul said, "I press toward the mark for the prize of the high calling of God in Christ Jesus" (Philippians 3:14, KJV).

Paul had a goal and he was relentless in his pursuit of it. He said, **"I press!"**

Pilgrims, you must daily press and pursue your goal to be healthy. There will be critics, haters, tempters, and those who think you are crazy.

Ignore them and **press on!**

Here is an acrostic that I like to use to help me keep having SUCCESS!

Pilgrims, in order to succeed you must:

See your goal.
Understand the obstacles.
Create a positive, mental picture.
Clear your mind of self-doubt.
Embrace the challenge.
Stay on track.
Show your loved ones you can do this.

Ask yourself how badly you really want to regain your health.

So many begin this journey, but few complete it because of a lack of **focus** and **determination**. Sadly, they will take two steps forward and three steps backward.

I am so glad that Jesus was focused and determined to accomplish His goal.

"He **steadfastly** set His face to go to Jerusalem" (Luke 9:51, KJV. See also Isaiah 50:7).

He would not be detoured. His concentration on the mission at hand could not be broken.

He was determined to succeed. His mind was made up!

How about you?

Press on, Pilgrims, and **patiently persevere** until you reach the peak of your mountain.

Then, shout as loud as you can with your hands raised high, "Praise God and the Lamb forevermore! **I DID IT!"**

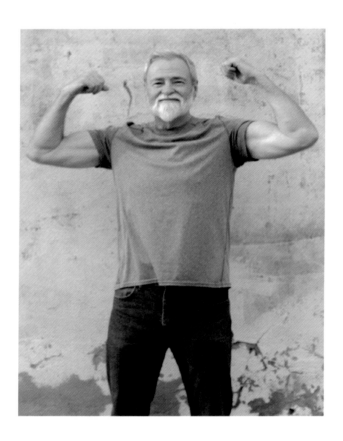

CHAPTER NINETEEN

MY APPEAL TO YOU...

"I will not die; instead, I will live
to tell what the Lord has done"
(Psalm 118:17, NLT).

Pilgrims, six years ago I was 80 pounds overweight. I was a walking time bomb, my blood pressure was so high I could have suffered a stroke or heart attack at any moment.

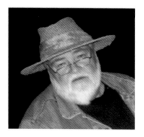 I was also pre-diabetic. I was always tired and just getting by, while I performed the normal responsibilities of a pastor, such as daily prayer, Bible study, and visitation to the hospital and nursing home.

My memory was slipping. I could no longer recall the names of people of classmates or fellow-workers from decades ago. It was always, "Hi, Bud," or "How are you doing, partner?" It was embarrassing, but I just thought it was normal for a man my age even though many of them could remember my name.

My father passed away at 57 from cancer, and my mother died at 62 from a stroke. I was 65 and had outlived both of them. I thought I was doing pretty well. The truth is I was not doing well at all. I had no vision for the church I was pastoring. I was just biding my time and going through the motions. I was getting by one day at a time and that was all. I wanted to finish my ministry and cross the finish line in a sprint. Truth is I could barely walk a short distance without being exhausted! Health issues were greatly hindering my ability to be all I wanted to be as a pastor, husband, father and grandfather. In my heart I knew this, but I was in denial. I was in trouble and needed help! On that wonderful Christmas Day of 2011, my son knew I needed help and gave me a book that transformed my life. It was as if he was throwing me a lifeline, knowing I was sinking fast. I grabbed hold of that line just in time. I was given an extension of life.

Perhaps you too will throw a lifeline to someone you love by giving him or her a copy of this book you are now reading!

When my wife insisted I go with her to the health fair at our local hospital, I didn't want to go. I thought it was just a waste of time. I was just a normal overweight pastor with no serious health concerns. **What a wake-up call I received!**

I was faced with a tough decision. Do I take the nurse's advice and go immediately to a doctor and begin taking blood pressure medicines? I have always believed, as a Christian, in seeking the counsel of the Lord. It was in prayer that I felt led to read that book my son had given me at Christmas.

This led to me reading over 80 other books on the topic of health and wellness, and reading countless medical studies.

The rest is history. The Lord, through prayer and the guidance of that book, has made it possible for me to say in the words of the Psalmist, "I will not die, I will live to tell what the Lord has done" (Psalm 118:17, NLT).

My wife and I celebrated our fifty-second wedding anniversary this year. I am blessed and thankful to be alive.

My heart is heavy and sad for the millions of Christian brothers and sisters who are in the same sinking boat I was in six years ago. Thankfully, in God's providential watch and care, **a lifeline was given to me.**

The Bible says this about Jesus' approach to Jerusalem that final week: "And when He was come near, He beheld the city, and wept over it" (Luke 19:41, KJV). It broke his heart, knowing their spiritual condition. He could save them, but only if they believed his message. "He that hath ears to hear let him hear" (Mark 4:9, KJV). This same verse in the New Living Translation says, "Anyone with ears to hear should listen and understand."

I see obese and overweight people each day, just like I used to be and I know that many of them are just as sick as I was. Two out of three people in America need the knowledge this book contains to regain their health.

Coupled with prayer, this knowledge can save millions of lives, but only if it is believed and put into practice.

Fellow pilgrims, my appeal to you is to live and not die.

Do not accept your present physical condition as normal. It is not normal for you to be sick, tired, and suffer from the side effects of prescription medications. The knowledge for your healing in this book is not esoteric, off the wall, bizarre, or weird.

You may believe it is very expensive to eat this way and that you have to eat grass-fed-only beef or pork. You may have heard that you must eat chickens and eggs that have been pasture-raised only. You may have heard that all your vegetables must be organic and come from your local farmer's market. All these things would be best, of course, but **they are not necessary in order to lose weight and regain your health.**

With the exception of local, free-range chicken eggs, all my food comes from our local grocery stores, and our food cost has gone down, not up.

Pilgrims, eating out is not a problem. My wife and I eat out at least once a week. **She has lost 36 pounds and no longer takes blood pressure medicine!** She was told she was a Type II Diabetic and was given Metformin, but she never took it. Now, her blood sugar is normal.

It was revealed in the news recently that Alzheimer's disease may be the third-leading cause of death in America, right behind cancer and heart disease. I may have been in the very early stages of Alzheimer's disease six years ago, but the ketogenic diet described in this book has reversed that. Alzheimer's is a disease of the mind that begins many years before the first symptoms appear.

My point is simple. If you have always eaten the Standard American Diet (SAD), you are at risk and should adopt the ketogenic diet immediately!

Your brain will thrive on ketones and is much less likely to develop Alzheimer's disease.

Your Commission

Pilgrims, chose to live fully!

Live for your spouse, children, and grandchildren.

Live for your neighbors and your church family.

Live for the Lord and, "see to it that you complete the ministry you received in the Lord" (Colossians 4:17, CEB).

Live and tell others what the Lord has done for you!

Pilgrims, what the good Lord has done for Patty and I, He will do for you! The information contained in this little book could save your life! Follow the path I have outlined here and you will regain your health.

Be aware that some of your friends will think you are crazy for following this plan, and actually wish you would change back to the way you were before. Misery loves company, you know.

Well, if you have some friends like that, I have a poem I want to share with you now...

When She Transformed Into a Butterfly,
The caterpillars spoke not of her beauty, but of her weirdness.
They wanted her to change back into what she always had been.
But she had wings.
Dean Jackson

Pilgrims, come along beside me and join me in dramatically improving the health of all Christians and further the work of God in this way!

"As iron sharpens iron, so a man sharpens the countenance of his friend" (Proverbs 27:17, NKJV).

Tell everyone you know about *The Pilgrim's Plan For Optimal Health!*

Your friend in Christ Jesus our Lord and Savior,

Pastor Dennis Burge

APPENDIXES

APPENDIX A

THE PILGRIM'S PLAN CLIFF NOTES

In the following section, I have distilled the Pilgrim's Plan down to the bare essentials. If you follow the recommendations in this section you will experience a dramatic increase in your health. I suggest you copy this list to a note card and tape on your bathroom mirror and your kitchen refrigerator. This gives you easy access to its wisdom.

THE PILGRIM'S NINE HACKS FOR FAST FAT LOSS

1. Eating fat is your best friend when it comes to losing fat. Real butter, coconut milk, coconut oil, MCT oil, extra virgin olive oil, heavy cream, nuts, seeds, avocados, and olives are all sources of good fats.

2. Eat protein in moderation, which is approximately your **goal** weight in grams, divided by .25.

Men's Example: 175-pound goal ÷.25 = 70 grams of protein per day.

Women's Example: 125-pound goal ÷.25 = 50 grams of protein per day.

NOTE: If you are very physically active, and you work out 3 or 4 times a week, or have a very physically challenging job, you need to add 50 percent more protein to these amounts in order to maintain your muscle mass.

3. Eat two meals per day, six hours apart. Intermittent fasting gives your body eighteen hours to burn fat as your primary fuel supply daily. However, if you are hungry between these two meals, eat a handful of nuts and drink a large glass of water.

4. Consume some Medium Chain Triglycerides (MCT) daily. MCT oil converts to ketone energy immediately and provides a high quality fat source that helps you maintain the proper macronutrient ratio that is necessary for dietary ketosis.

You can put MCT oil in your bulletproof coffee or tea first thing in the morning and again three hours later. Start with a teaspoon and work up to one tablespoon over time.

Remember, this is not regular coconut oil, but it will be labeled as MCT oil. There is a difference! This provides critical healthy fats for your diet. I use Now Foods brand MCT Oil.

If you don't want to use MCT Oil in your coffee or tea, follow the alternative and consume one to two tablespoons of regular Coconut Oil straight from the container per day. I use Barlean's brand because it has the best taste I've found.

For more information see Chapter Eleven and the section titled "Replace Your Breakfast With This...".

5. Drink lots of water, so that you stay well hydrated. Drink one cup of water a half hour before your meals. This also will help suppress your hunger before you eat. Drink very little water with your meals **so as not to dilute your digestive juices.**

6. Avocado is the healthiest fruit on earth. They are full of potassium, a critical electrolyte, and are a heart-healthy monounsaturated fat. Eat one or two per day and no other fruit until you've reached your goal. They are also very high in soluble fiber, which can help lower glucose levels.

7. Eat lots of vegetables that are non-starchy, low calorie, and high in fiber, vitamins, minerals, and antioxidants.

8. Coffee and tea are full of antioxidants that are very beneficial for optimal health, and caffeine will help you burn fat as well as energize you. However, too much will affect your ability to sleep properly at night. Therefore, I recommend you not consume any caffeine after midday.

9. Adequate sleep is critical to your success at losing weight/fat. I recommend seven to nine hours of sleep per day. A 15-minute power nap during the day will do wonders for everyone.

APPENDIX B

PILGRIM'S PLAN FOOD LIST

The lists below make up the foundation of my nutrition. I highly suggest during the period you are trying to lose weight that you stick to the foods on these pages. After you have reached your goal weight, you may experiment with other foods.

NINE FOOD GROUP RECOMMENDATIONS
1. Beef
2. Fowl
3. Fish
4. Pork
5. Eggs
6. Non-starchy vegetables
7. Fruit (only after you have reached your ideal weight)
8. Nuts and seeds
9. Collagen peptide protein powder and zero carb isolate protein powder

NON-STARCHY VEGETABLES RECOMMENDATIONS
Keep in mind there are many other choices you can make that are excellent. These are just my favorites.

1. Broccoli
2. Cauliflower
3. Mushrooms (shitake and portabella are my favorites, especially sautéed in real butter. KerryGold brand butter is my favorite.)

4. Spinach
5. Romaine lettuce
6. Green beans (the one exception to the bean rule)
7. Cucumbers
8. Brussels sprouts
9. Zucchini

GOOD, HEALTHY FATS RECOMMENDATIONS
1. Avocado
2. Butter
3. Extra virgin olive oil
4. Olives
5. Bacon drippings
6. Coconut oil
7. Coconut milk
8. Heavy cream
9. MCT oil

GUIDE TO NINE SUPER SPICES

As you begin to adopt the Pilgrim's Plan way of eating you will want to explore the rich and diverse spices that the good Lord has provided for us. Spices provide an added dimension to the foods we eat, can have specific health benefits, and are a wonderful way to make dishes come alive with flavor. In this appendix I've listed my top nine spices, but don't stop here! Please keep exploring and expanding your knowledge of how spices can improve the taste and enjoyment of your food.

Turmeric

This super spice helps control blood sugar and slows down the metabolism of carbohydrates after meals. It also helps prevent cancer by inhibiting the genetic switches that allow cancer cell growth. Turmeric increases cellular energy. It also removes plaque in the brain that can lead to Alzheimer's disease. It reduces inflammation and joint pain caused by arthritis.

Tarragon

Tarragon helps blood circulation and reduces plaque in the arteries. It also significantly lowers bad cholesterol and increases good cholesterol. Use one teaspoon a day and your heart will thank you.

Oregano

High in antioxidants and antibacterial compounds, it is very good in tomato dishes.

Bay leaf

Bay is a natural pain reliever. It is great in soups, stews, and pot roasts.

Rosemary

Rosemary improves memory just by smelling it and is very good on grilled meats.

Cayenne

Increases blood flow and metabolism. Sprinkle a little on about anything to add sweet heat.

Cinnamon

Helps control blood sugar levels and slow carbohydrate metabolism by up to 30 percent. Sprinkle a little on any vegetable for a sweet and savory delight!

Dill

Dill has antibacterial properties that kill intestinal bugs and reduces bloating. It is very good with fish and chicken.

Sage

Sage is a memory enhancer and great on pork dishes.

Note: I recommend you use fresh spices when possible and stay away from irradiated spices. Irradiation destroys the essential micronutrients that can help you reach optimal health.

APPENDIX D

REFERENCES AND RESEARCH SOURCES

During my research for this book, I read over 80 books and read many scientific studies in order to ensure that The Pilgrim's Plan was on the cutting edge of nutritional science. I owe a great debt of gratitude to each of the authors and researchers for their fine work and inspiration.

However, during my research, I came across many opinions that differ from the Biblical account of creation. I believe the Bible account of the genesis of all things. This includes the creation, not the evolution, of mankind. If anything, I believe that man has not evolved, he has devolved.

When reading any secular writing, you must always use your gift of discernment. Do not throw the baby out with the bathwater of evolutionary teaching, which is contained in many of the books listed here.

Physically speaking, there is life-saving information contained within these books. As a Christian, you have the spirit of discernment (see 1 Corinthians 12:10) within you to filter out the vile from the precious (see Jeremiah 15:19).

I have listed my top reference books plus my favorite website on the next page.

"I sincerely believe the Keto Reset diet could represent the greatest breakthrough in the history of nutritional science and the history of dieting to promote successful long-term fat loss and weight management" Mark Sission

1. *The Keto Reset Diet.* Mark Sisson with Brad Kearns
2. *The Art and Science of Low Carbohydrate Performance.* Jeff S. Volek, PhD, RD, Stephen D. Phinney, MD, PhD
3. *The Art and Science of Low Carbohydrate Living.* Jeff S. Volek, PhD, RD and Stephen D. Phinney, MD, PhD
4. *Primal Fat Burner.* Nora T. Gedgaudas, CNS, CNT
5. *Primal Body, Primal Mind.* Nora T. Gedgaudas, CNS, CNT
6. *Fat For Fuel.* Dr. Joseph Mercola
7. *Why We Get Fat.* and *Good Calories, Bad Calories* Gary Taubes
8. *Wheat Belly.* William Davis, MD
9. *Grain Brain.* David Perlmutter, MD
10. *The Big Fat Surprise.* Nina Teicholz
11. *Keto Zone Diet.* Don Colbert, MD
12. *Keto.* Maria Emmerich-Craig
13. *The Bulletproof Diet.* Dave Asprey
14. *The Paleo Solution.* Robb Wolf
15. *The Obesity Epidemic.* Zoe Harcombe, BA, MA
16. *It Starts With Food.* Dallas and Melissa Hartwig
17. *Headstrong.* Dave Asprey
18. *The Primal Blueprint 21 Day Total Body Transformation.* Mark Sisson (This is the book my son gave me!)
19. *Dr. Bernstein's Diabetes Solution.* Richard K. Bernstien, MD
20. *The New Primal Blueprint* Mark Sisson
21. *Practical Paleo.* Diane Sanfilippo, BS, NC
22. *The Ketogenic Diet.* Kristen Mancinelli, MS, RD
23. *The end of Alzheimer's.* Dale E.Bredesen,M.D.
24. *Ketogenic Bible* Dr. Jacob Wilson & Ryan Lowery
25. *The Paleo Thyroid Solution* Elle Russ & Gary E Forseman, MD
26. *The Case Against Sugar* Gary Taubes
27. *The Alzheimer's Antidote* Amy Berger, MS, CNS, NTP
28. *The World Turned Upside Down* Dr. David Feinman, Ph. D
29. www.marksdailyapple.com

ANNOUNCING THE
PILGRIM'S PLAN COOKBOOK!

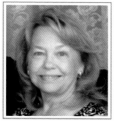 One of the biggest requests we get is for help with recipes and meal planning. To meet this need we have created an invaluable resource for anyone implementing the Pilgrim's Plan.

The Pilgrim's Plan Cookbook is full of over 80 recipes that have been created, cooked, and enjoyed in our family for years.

These recipes were the key to Dennis and I regaining our health and we want you to have access to them!

You see, for as long as I can remember, I have been addicted to sugar and carbs. I didn't know it, but it was a fact.

As a child I enjoyed copious amounts of desserts. There were always peanut butter or oatmeal cookies, chocolate cake, cobblers, and strawberry shortcake when the berries were in season. I couldn't wait to get to the cupcakes and mints at baby showers and birthday parties.

My breakfast consisted of Cheerios with plenty of sugar or a cup of sweet hot chocolate and several pieces of toast.

I went to school feeling slightly nauseated a lot of mornings. I was always low energy, and didn't know why. Even as an adult it was hard for me to wake up in the mornings, and I felt foggy-headed for most of the day.

My sisters and I would talk about our lack of alertness but we had no solutions to offer one another.

In spite of all this, I was always petite…until our 4th son was born. Then, I steadily gained weight over the years until my 4'11" frame was carrying 145 pounds!

By that time I had developed osteoarthritis, which was becoming more and more painful and obvious. It was getting difficult to bend to reach items in my lower cabinets or on the floor. I became winded while climbing stairs or walking an incline.

In addition, I had acid reflux and had to keep antacids within reach at all times. I awakened every night with heartburn and had to take medicine for the burning sensation. Eventually, I began investing in Prilosec on a regular basis. I was just generally uncomfortable and unhappy with my physical condition.

After visiting a clinic for a general wellness check I received a letter from the doctor, explaining her findings.

I had been taking a prescription blood pressure medication for several years. But now, it seemed that I was facing another health issue.

The words on that letter jumped out at me and shocked me to my core:

"YOU ARE NOW DIABETIC."

I can't tell you why I was so surprised. I should have known. I was eating all the carbs and sugar I wanted. There was no limit.

And I was steadily putting on the weight.

At first, as I looked at those black words on white paper, I thought, "This isn't me. I can't be diabetic!"

There was no diabetes in my immediate family, but I had heard the stories about my husband's grandmother, who was so ill with it that she lost a leg to the disease, and not long after that she passed away.

Until my weight and blood pressure climbed, I had been healthy all of my life. The thought of living with this diagnosis was frightening, to say the least.

At first I felt helpless, then I became a little angry with myself for allowing this to happen to me.

Deep down, I had known that my body would not tolerate the abuse I was giving it on a daily basis, and yet, it took a crisis to get me to make a change.

I am so thankful that the change was a few simple, dietary adjustments. Yes, it took some willpower and some learning, but the alternative was not acceptable to me.

About this same time, my husband had a similar experience with his health issues. He began to read, research, and learn all he could about high blood pressure and diabetes, and the effects of our diets on these, as well as other diseases. The Pilgrim's Plan is the result of his studies.

Meanwhile, the doctor prescribed Metformin for me to control the Type II Diabetes.

I had the prescription filled, but I knew I was never going to take it. If sugar and carbs had put me in this condition, I figured that controlling my consumption of these would at least help reverse it, and I might lose a few pounds along the way.

Together, Dennis and I ditched the sugary, carb-laden desserts. We omitted starchy vegetables and sugary drinks from our table as well.

I was amazed to learn that good food is good medicine.

I was equally shocked to learn that the food pyramid is all wrong.

Most importantly, I learned that we can eat well without indulging in foods that could ultimately make us sick and possibly shorten our lives.

After a short time I gradually reduced the blood pressure medicine until I was able to stop taking it altogether and my blood sugar normalized.

I began to lose the weight and shed 36 pounds in about 7 months.

I have abundant energy and the foggy-headed feeling that I was plagued with has disappeared.

I feel alert all day and my ability to concentrate has improved.

I don't hurt from arthritis, as I once did, which makes a lot of difference in my quality of life.

The eradication of heartburn and acid reflux has been miraculous.

This was almost immediate, and it was the first benefit of our change of diet. Both my husband and I were able to throw out our supplies of antacids.

I have always cooked, ever since my husband taught me how to scramble eggs. I had never cooked a meal when we got married, but soon learned that I was going to have to step up to the plate...so to speak.

We raised 4 sons and I have always enjoyed impressing them and their families with family meals around the table. It has been a real challenge for me to change most of what I know, to what is better.

Ingredients are different, but better.

Results are different, but better.

I never imagined that I would produce a cookbook, much less one that didn't include sugar and white flour. If anyone had told me that I could make a delicious carrot cake with cream cheese frosting, without flour and sugar, I would have argued that it couldn't be done.

I began cooking, the Pilgrim's way, gradually and with simple recipes. I learned how to use sugar-free sweeteners to produce amazing desserts, and I learned how to thicken gravies and sauces without flour or cornstarch.

I would like this cookbook to encourage you, to help you transition to a healthier way of cooking and eating, to a healthier lifestyle. All my recipes are low carb and sugar free.

Soon, you will be converting some of your own recipes to a healthier version. If you have a failure, try again and don't be discouraged.

As you get started, I have a few words of encouragement and wisdom I'd like to share. When beginning this lifestyle it can be a little daunting. Going through the recipes, you will see ingredients that you are not familiar with... things that sound strange.

I understand because I have been where you are.

I thought I could never make the transition to healthy cooking because I had cooked the traditional way for my whole adult life.

It was only after I personally realized the health benefits of omitting white flour, sugar and most processed foods from my diet that I became committed to the change.

Don't think that you have to clean out your cupboards immediately and completely re-stock.

Start with the basic recipes. Add new, healthy ingredients to your shopping list and your pantry will soon be full of healthy, nutritious foods. Most items I use can be bought at my local big box store.

I do like to shop at the larger food club stores and buy in bulk when I can. They help cut costs on many items such as almond flour, nuts, cream cheese etc.

And don't be afraid to experiment and change any recipe to your liking. Get creative! Most importantly, know that

I am always here to help if you have questions!

To get your personal copy of the Pilgrim's Plan cook book, please go to www.pilgrimsplan.com to order one for you, and one for a friend!

Patty Burge

Patty Burge
Creator of the Pilgrim's Plan Cookbook
March 2017

Interested? Here's a sample of some of our delicious meals highlighted in the cookbook. These amazing recipies developed by me and my husband transformed our lives and restored our health.

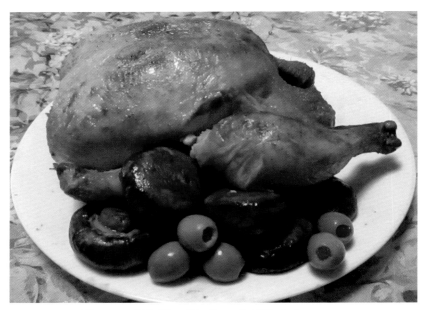

Beautifully Baked Chicken

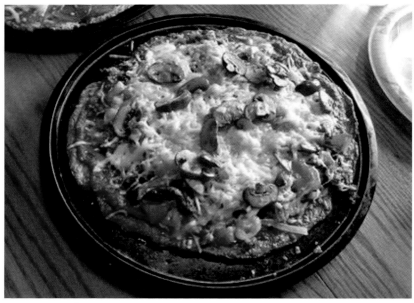

Cheese Lover's Pizza Your Way

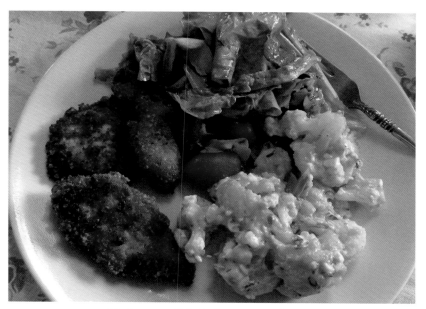

Crispy Chicken Strips

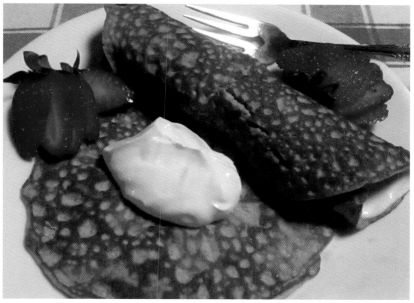

Cream Cheese Pancakes

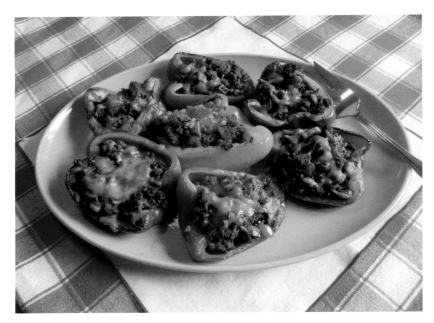

Taco Stuffed Peppers

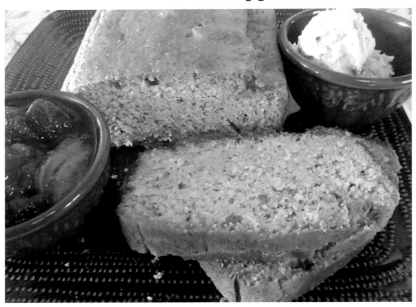

Keto Coconut Bread Loaf

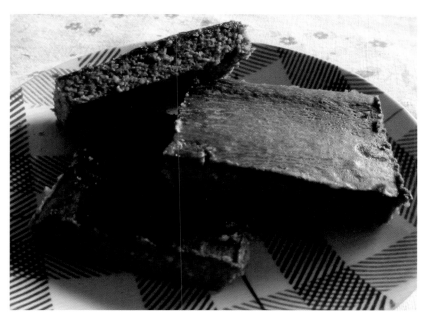

Decadent Chocolate Sheet Cake

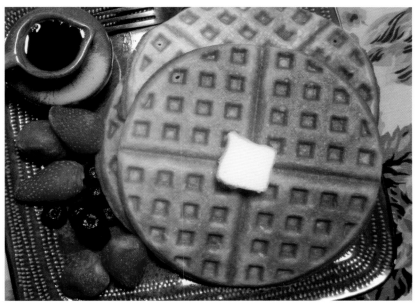

Waffles Keto Style

JOIN THE
COMMUNITY OF PILGRIMS
TODAY!

The Community of Pilgrims is where we share many additional benefits with our community on how to implement the Pilgrim's Plan most effectively.

If you are serious about achieving optimal health and wellness, then you will want to be part of this dynamic group, which is free to join as part of your purchase of this book!

Inside the Community Of Pilgrims, we will...

- Release new Pilgrim's Plan approved recipes, meal plans and shopping lists!

- Answer all your questions and provide additional guidance.

- Have special member-only promotions!

- Recognize our members and share success stories.

- Post new inspiring articles and research studies.

Come be part of the family and enjoy getting to know the other Pilgrims on the same journey as YOU!

Sign up at
www.facebook.com/groups/communityofpilgrims